EDWARD JARVIS
and the Medical World
of Nineteenth-Century America

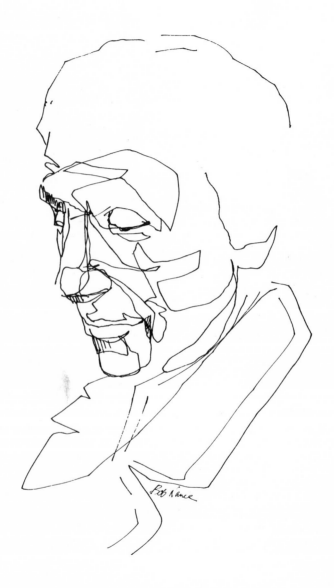

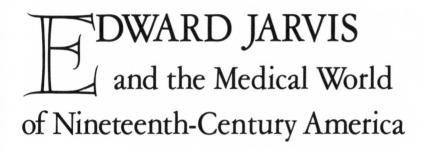

EDWARD JARVIS
and the Medical World
of Nineteenth-Century America

Gerald N. Grob

THE UNIVERSITY OF TENNESSEE PRESS
KNOXVILLE

Frontispiece: Line drawing of Edward Jarvis, about 1870, from an original likeness, courtesy of Harvard Medical School Library

Library of Congress Cataloging in Publication Data

Grob, Gerald N   1931–
   Edward Jarvis and the medical world of nineteenth-
century America.

   Bibliography: p.
   Includes index.
   1. Jarvis, Edward, 1803–1884. 2. Psychiatrists—
United States—Biography. 3. Medicine—United States
—History—19th century. I. Title.
RC339.52.J37G76   616.8'9'00924 [B]   78–3771
ISBN 0–87049–239–X

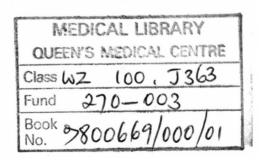

FOR *Bradford, Evan, and Seth*

Preface

M ore than fifteen years ago I first encountered the name of Edward Jarvis. As my research on the history of American psychiatry and mental hospitals progressed, I began to realize that Jarvis, despite his relative obscurity, was a significant figure whose interests and concerns covered a variety of subjects, including psychiatry, public health, statistical inquiry, and social policy. An accidental discovery of his hitherto unknown letter books resulted in this biography.

As I pursued Jarvis through his long career, it became increasingly clear that his conceptions of medicine, society, and disease were so interrelated that it was impossible to deal with one without touching upon the others. Nor could his commitment to medicine be understood without reference to the larger religious, intellectual, and cultural milieu of which he was a part. It was also abundantly clear that many of the generalizations about medicine, the medical profession, and social policy and social thought left much to be desired. For example, the familiar categories used by historians—conservative and liberal—made little sense when applied to mid-nineteenth-century America. My goal in undertaking this study, therefore, was to attempt to re-create as accurately as possible the life of an individual whose training and outlook reflected a variety of social, intellectual, religious, scientific, and economic currents.

Much to my surprise, I found that beneath Jarvis's varied and seemingly compartmentalized activities lay a unified and coherent set of beliefs that gave meaning to his life and also helped to illuminate the theory and practice of mid-nineteenth-century medicine. Like countless other human beings, Jarvis spent most of his adult life in an effort to reconcile traditional beliefs with those impersonal forces that were leading his country into the modern world. Indeed, many of the problems for which he sought answers continue to be of concern; social change and scientific advance have not always been synonymous with progress.

During the preparation of this book I have drawn upon many persons for aid. In particular, I should like to thank George A. Billias, Philip Greven, Richard Kohn, Jacques Quen, Barbara G. Rosenkrantz, and the late George Rosen, all of whom gave me the benefit of their time and knowledge. I should also like to express my deep appreciation to Richard J. Wolfe of the Countway Library of Medicine of the Harvard Medical School, who provided the kind of assistance that only historians can understand, and the staff of the Rutgers University Library, who always responded to my requests with graciousness and cooperation. A grant from the Public Health Service, National Library of Medicine (HEW), No. 2306, greatly facilitated the research and writing without in any way infringing upon the freedom of the investigator. A fellowship from the National Endowment for the Humanities also provided a leave during the early stages of this project. Above all, I should like to acknowledge a debt that I owe to my wife, Lila K. Grob, that can never be adequately repaid. She aided me in ways too numerous to list, and provided the encouragement that led me to persevere.

New Brunswick, N.J.   GERALD N. GROB
October 1977

Contents

EDWARD JARVIS
and the Medical World
of Nineteenth-Century America

Introduction

During the nineteenth century the theory and practice of medicine in the United States and Europe underwent sharp changes. Before 1800 the overwhelming majority of physicians were concerned more with the treatment than the prevention of disease. After 1800, on the other hand, concern with the prevention of disease became more significant as the medical profession confronted a number of pressing intellectual and scientific issues. What was the function of medicine if traditional practice did not result in demonstrable cures? What was the nature and origin of disease? Admittedly, the typical practitioner immersed in the day-to-day treatment of individual patients cared little for such abstractions. But to a much smaller group of individuals sensitive to and aware of contemporary intellectual, scientific, and social currents, these questions could not be so easily dismissed. In their efforts to grapple with them they slowly began to redefine the foundation of their profession and to create a different theoretical framework that involved subtle shifts in their role and status. The proper function of medicine, they proclaimed, was to prevent disease by specifying those social and environmental conditions that promoted the maintenance of health; a true physician was at the same time a social activist and educator.

The changes that overtook medicine after 1800 resulted from the convergence of several developments. The rise of taxonomical botany in the eighteenth century contributed to the growing medical fascination with nosography and nosology. In the succeeding century considerable effort went into the development of elaborate classifications of disease, partly under the belief that to classify was to understand. As nosology became more important, the stage was set for an emphasis on the systematic collection of aggregate data. Concern with such data, of course, was not new. The rise of the nation-state earlier had set the stage for the emergence of "political arithmetic" by such figures as William Petty and John Graunt, both of whom were keenly aware of the relationship between a healthy and growing population on the one hand and national power and prestige on the other. The result was a growing interest in a social analysis based on the use of aggregate data. By the eighteenth century many European states were collecting population and mortality statistics, a development that would help to reshape medicine in the nineteenth century. Indeed, the basic problem after 1800 was to collect data and to define appropriate categories. The ever-growing concern with national power, coupled with the newer social problems related to modernization, provided an appropriate environment for the mature development of a system that held out the promise of providing solutions to problems involving morbidity and mortality.

In the United States the growing importance of taxonomy and quantification was reinforced by indigenous developments. During the first half of the nineteenth century most institutions of higher learning were under the influence of Scottish Common Sense philosophy or—as it was called—moral philosophy. In reaction to Hume's devastating skepticism, moral philosophers attempted to strengthen the foundations of Protestant Christianity by reasserting the lawful and moral nature of the universe and the rational nature of mankind. An important by-product of their efforts was a renewed faith in Baconian science with its emphasis on the collection of particular facts and the derivation of general laws from these facts. In turn Baconian science made possible the rapid acceptance of a statistically oriented social research which emerged from the work of figures like Adolphe Quetelet, who developed a method based on the assumption that social changes would be accompanied by corresponding changes in statistical averages. Those physicians who would help to reshape their profession came from a milieu dominated by moral philosophy and a Baconian view of science. Disillusionment with traditional therapeutics and concepts of disease by the 1820s and 1830s also reinforced the conviction that new approaches were necessary. The findings of the Paris school in particular helped to discredit traditional therapeutics. By the second third of the nineteenth century the stage was set for the emergence of a new approach that would alter traditional medical concepts and establish new roles for physicians.

Finally, most practitioners had direct contact with the problems that accompanied rapid industrial and population growth. Their perceptions of existing social and economic problems helped to condition and to shape their views about health, disease, and mortality. Indeed, the medical world of mid-nineteenth-century America was but a mirror of the problems and divisions that seemed to threaten the unity and homogeneity of the larger society; medical debates over normative standards of health and behavior corresponded to other more general debates that dealt with the future of a nation.

The younger activists who reached professional maturity in the 1830s and 1840s were, unlike their predecessors, concerned primarily with the maintenance of health. Influenced as much by their moral and religious beliefs as their scientific training, they defined health in terms of a proper and symbiotic relationship between nature, society, and the individual. Convinced that a divine power had created a universe governed by immutable natural law, they interpreted disease and social evil as the results of unlawful (or immoral) behavior. Mortality patterns—like crime rates—were a true measure of the moral fiber of a society. The role of the physician was twofold: to discover those individual and social factors governing health and to disseminate those findings among their fellow countrymen in order that they be put to practical use. In their eyes medicine was inseparably linked with social policy; as such the profession occupied a strategic position in a society facing all of the problems arising out of urbanization, economic change, and immigration. Whether dealing with poverty, disease, mortality, nutritional patterns, crime, or environmental pollution, their message was consistent; individuals and society had within reach the power to alter those conditions that resulted in disease and premature mortality. The medical profession, therefore, had a crucial part to play in the task of social regeneration.

Such convictions led physicians and other like-minded individuals down hitherto ignored paths. Some would seek to alter the quality of urban life by promoting better housing, clean water, and unadulterated and pure food; some would become involved in crusades against the use of alcohol and tobacco; some would fight for free universal education; some would devote their energies to furthering the movement to collect accurate vital statistics in order to illuminate the conditions of life and death, health and disease; and some would fight for the establishment of institutions to provide care and treatment for a variety of distressed groups, such as the poor, the infirm, the aged, the sick, the insane, the criminal, and the juvenile orphan and delinquent.

Curiously enough, many of these physicians and activists harbored ambivalent feelings. They shared a sense of optimism about the future; science and philanthropy made possible the creation of a good and harmonious social order. But they feared that the immoral and unlawful behavior of undesirable groups threatened the very fabric of American society. Their analyses and programs, therefore, often reflected both pessimism and optimism. Disagreeing on many specific issues, they nevertheless remained united in their belief that individual and social perfection lay within reach of all human beings.

In many urban communities such physicians functioned as important members of local elites. Their elevated status was not a function of their earning capacity; better opportunities existed in other occupations. Nor was their status a function of their ability to restrict entry into the profession; before and after 1830 there were virtually no barriers to the right to practice medicine. On the contrary, status was a function of the profession's very perception of disease. For if disease was a function of individual and social factors, then the services provided by the medical profession were of inestimable value to the community that could not be expressed merely in economic terms. Physicians, like clergymen, played a variety of roles; both ministered to man's spiritual and physical needs and served as sure moral guides. The true physician was a philanthropist and social activist by nature; diagnosis, prognosis, and treatment alone could not justify the raison d'etre of the profession.[1]

Assuredly, the individuals who helped to forge a new synthesis that would briefly define the essential character of American medicine between 1840 and 1870 disagreed among themselves as often as they agreed. Some advocated a powerful interventionist government to deal with social and medical problems; others saw the salvation of society in terms of individual redemption. But for the most part their disagreements were over specific issues; on basic assumptions they remained united.

Today relatively little is known about the careers of those who shaped the theory and practice of medicine in mid-nineteenth-century America, partly because their approach was quickly overwhelmed in the 1880s and afterward by the specific germ theory of disease and a technology that altered medical practice. The names of figures like John H. Griscom, Edwin M. Snow, Edward Barton, Elisha Harris, Wilson Jewell, and Henry G. Clark remain for the most part unknown. Much the same holds true for Edward Jarvis. Yet from the 1840s to the 1870s Jarvis was a figure of considerable eminence. He ranked among the leading three or four American psychiatrists of that period; his *Report on Insanity* to the Massachusetts legislature in 1855 was the most significant statistical social survey of that malady in the nineteenth century. But like innumerable others of that generation, Jarvis did not confine his efforts to a single problem. The process of specialization had not yet transformed medicine, and the line between professional competence and general service was as yet vague or nonexistent. Consequently, Jarvis was a contributor to and publicist for the young public health movement; he helped to lay the foundations of the modern federal census as a source of data and an instrument of policy; he stimulated the movement to record and to preserve vital statistics in order to shed light on the conditions of health and disease; and he wrote extensively on social and medical issues.

Like others of his generation, Jarvis was concerned with the scope and implications of rapid social and economic change. What was the relationship between urbanization and morbidity and mortality patterns? Could the pressures of a competitive and business-oriented society explain the wide prevalence of mental disease? Did immigration of lower-class groups with different cultural and religious patterns threaten the well-being of the American people? Were there differences in the behavioral patterns of male and female? What were the sources of such varied social problems as disease, premature mortality, and even crime? Above all, what constituted appropriate responses to critical social problems that threatened to alter the character of American society?

In seeking answers to such questions, Jarvis did not begin with a completely uncommitted or neutral mind. On the contrary, his perceptions of the world were already partly conditioned by his early upbringing and education in a family and community that shared a coherent set of beliefs about the orderly nature of the universe and the existence of eternal moral values. In his later career he would repeatedly seek to fuse these moral preconceptions with the data derived from scientific and medical research. In so doing he would contribute to the creation of a new intellectual and scientific synthesis that would reshape the theory and practice of medicine and move it in the direction of the emerging social sciences. To be sure, developments after 1870 fragmented the fragile alliance between medical and social science; each would follow very different paths in the succeeding century. Nevertheless, the issues posed by Jarvis and others of his generation were sufficiently important that neither the contemporary medical profession nor the academic disciplines that make up the social and behavioral sciences have been able to dismiss or to ignore them.

1

The Making of a Physician

Lewis Mumford once compared nineteenth-century Concord with the vitality and cultural unity of fifth-century Athens, thirteenth-century Florence, and sixteenth-century London. No doubt Mumford's ranking of this small Massachusetts community was somewhat exaggerated. Yet to many the town more than merited its accolades. It was the scene of the first military engagement of the American Revolution, an event, to quote Timothy Dwight, that changed human affairs, altered the balance of human power, and introduced "a new direction to the course of human improvement. Man, from the events which have occurred here, will in some respects assume a new character, and experience in some respects a new destiny."[1]

Certainly the first half of the nineteenth century seemed to fulfill Dwight's expectations. Although the population of Concord did not reach two thousand until about 1830, it was already becoming an attraction to a group of young intellectuals. At one time or another the town would boast of having as its residents Ralph Waldo Emerson, Henry David Thoreau, Bronson Alcott, George W. Curtis, and Nathaniel Hawthorne, to mention only a few. Some nineteenth-century observers might have added Edward Jarvis to this list. To our generation, however, his inclusion would cause perplexity, if only because of the obscurity of his name and career. Yet to his contemporaries Jarvis was a figure of considerable eminence; his reputation extended beyond the borders of his native land.

I

Edward Jarvis, the fourth of seven children of Francis Jarvis and Millicent Hosmer, was born in Concord on January 9, 1803.

Originally from Normandy, the Jarvis family had migrated first to England and then to the American colonies in the seventeenth century. Edward's grandfather, John Jarvis, was one of those unsuccessful entrepreneurs forever seeking but never finding his fortune. In 1765 he married Elizabeth Bowman, and between 1767 and 1784 the couple had nine children. Still hoping to improve himself, John Jarvis temporarily left his family and moved to western New York in 1785. Shortly thereafter he died from some unknown disease. Lacking resources, his widow was forced to place the children who were able to work with families who could provide them with the opportunity of earning a living.[2]

Edward's father, Francis Jarvis, was the second oldest son. Following his father's death, he went to live with a Mr. Richardson of Watertown. There he became friendly with Richardson's son John, from whom he learned the bakery trade. Without formal education, Francis nevertheless possessed considerable ambition and drive as well as a thirst for knowledge. His lack of schooling proved no impediment, and he became well versed in such academic subjects as mathematics, geography, and history. In 1789 he moved with the Richardsons to Concord, a town whose citizens had begun to experience a commercial boom following the signing of the treaty of peace with England in 1783. There he worked in Richardson's tavern and supervised the house. The following year Francis entered into a partnership with Thomas Safford and together they opened a bakehouse. The business proved profitable and after five years Francis was able to buy out his partner and later acquire a farm. In 1793 he married Millicent Hosmer, a sixth-generation American from an old and prominent Concord family, a step that enhanced his standing in the community. Their first son Francis was born the following year; the others followed at roughly two-year intervals. The second and sixth were daughters, one of whom died at the age of three and the other at sixteen. Altogether five sons survived in the Jarvis household; Francis, Jr., and Charles were the two older brothers, Edward the middle, and Stephen and Nathan the younger. Relatively successful in business, Francis Jarvis quickly became one of the pillars of the community. In 1798 he joined the Concord Social Circle, an organization devoted to the preservation of the memories of all of its members. In 1810 he became a member of Ezra Ripley's Congregational Church; two years later he was elected deacon, a position that he held until his death in 1840. In addition, he served on the school committee for many years.[3]

The household in which young Edward grew to maturity was patriarchal in nature. The father was clearly the dominant figure and influence upon the children. Edward once noted that there was "nothing remarkable" about his mother. His descriptions of his father were far more vibrant in tone and suggest that their relationship might have had elements of competition or hostility. His father, wrote Edward, held notions of morality that were "rigid to the extreme" even though he was Arminian in his religious views. While tempering an austere and firm rule with affection and love, he taught his children to respect authority, order, and virtue. It was hardly surprising that, holding such opinions, he was a Federalist rather than a Republican in his politics. But the intense political strife that strained relationships elsewhere and encouraged bitter conflict was not characteristic of Concord, and Francis remained on good terms even with those who did not share his views.[4]

Edward's childhood was relatively uneventful. Although he never outwardly rejected parental authority, the surviving sources suggest that his obedient exterior concealed a streak of resentment toward his father. Yet he never questioned his father's concept of an orderly and hierarchical universe governed by immutable moral laws that prescribed proper modes of conduct and behavior; in many ways the son and father had similar personalities and beliefs. With most of his brothers Edward developed close ties. He was most intimate with Charles, who was just two years his senior. His relationship with Francis Jr., the eldest, was never close, for Edward found him to be an "unsociable person" usually immersed in his own affairs.[5]

The town of Concord further strengthened his sense of living in a closely knit community. Founded in 1635, the town was located nearly twenty miles west of Boston. Its growth was slow: in 1765 the population was just under 1,600, and a century later it still contained only slightly over 2,200 people. More than anything else, the American Revolution gave Concord its sense of self-identity; few residents could forget the battle that launched that struggle. The growing material prosperity that became evident in the decade after the Revolution further reinforced the confidence of its inhabitants, and, as Jarvis recalled in later life, strengthened an already well-developed sense of community cohesiveness. Although Jarvis spent most of his adult career elsewhere, he never ceased to long for the town in which he had been born and had grown to maturity; in his old age he devoted his final decade to gathering materials for its history.[6]

Like other Bay State communities, Concord prized education, a fact that was reflected in the relatively large number of local residents who graduated from Harvard College. Edward attended the town schools almost continuously to the age of fourteen. His father's faith in the value of education—a faith that led him to collect an unusually large personal library of about 250 volumes—no doubt influenced his son's receptivity toward schooling. Edward learned grammar at seven, arithmetic at eleven, and geometry, trigonometry, and surveying at thirteen. Even during these early years he acquired a considerable reputation for his mathematical achievements, a trait that would help to shape his future career.[7]

Edward's character was further molded by the religious milieu of his youth. Although conflict over theological issues was by no means absent from Concord during the seventeenth and eighteenth centuries, an era of religious stability was inaugurated with the selection of Ezra Ripley as pastor in 1778. Ripley, a Harvard graduate, was then twenty-seven years of age. His ministry in Concord was to last sixty-three years, terminating only with his death in 1841. A less than profound thinker, Ripley derived his influence more from his amiable and friendly character and length in office than from his learning or knowledge. In his eyes Christianity was an eminently practical religion that provided a sure guide to life and morality. Given such views, it was hardly surprising that Ripley and his church eventually rejected the Trinitarian position and became Unitarian.[8]

Few children who grew up in Concord during these decades could have avoided Ripley, and Edward was no exception. There was little doubt of the child's warm feelings; all of Edward's later reminiscences refer to Ripley in kind and admiring terms. Between his father's influence on the one side and Dr. Ripley's on the other, Jarvis may have developed a dislike of theological conflict over abstract religious doctrines. This is not in any way to imply that religion was an insignificant element in his life. On the contrary, the very opposite was true. He could not help but see the world in terms of Protestant and especially Unitarian Christianity. He had few doubts about the existence of God or the moral character of the universe. Heir to the revolt against the Calvinist view that salvation was conferred upon sinful human beings by a mysterious and arbitrary Deity, Edward preferred to think of God as a creator and governor who followed the laws of physics that He originally created. Jarvis's view of religion led unerringly in an activist direction. Sin was due to the selfish but voluntary actions of individuals. Right and wrong were clearly distinguishable, and all human beings had the freedom to choose between them. From these beliefs he drew the corollary that humanity, as it gradually acquired knowledge, wisdom, and understanding, could deal more effectively with its ills and problems. In this respect he shared the optimism, faith in progress, and belief in perfectionism so characteristic of antebellum America. A full understanding of natural law was the means by which mankind could resolve age-old problems and ultimately create a better world. "I have no faith nor desire for religion further than it makes me better," Jarvis confided in his diary in early 1828.

Of itself, it is nothing, its effects alone are what I think desirable. I do not wish to build up a system mysterious & separate from common life. I only wish it to apply to every thing I do or say or think, to govern my thoughts words & actions according to the eternal principles of truth, the will of God, & when the soul be separated from the body, I believe the former will have a power of reflection to the sinner, bitter, galling and a hell; to the virtuous man a source of unending delight, a Heaven.

This is my religion. Of what I believe I will not now say, thinking it is of less consequence what a man believes than what he does & from what motives. If these last two are good, it is well, if not, woe be unto him.[9]

II

At the age of fourteen Edward began to help his father in the bake house and on the farm, attending school about two-thirds of the year. By the time he reached fifteen there was some question about his future. He disliked his father's business, preferring instead to attend college or to enter a mercantile occupation. The first alternative seemed improbable, since Charles was already attending Harvard College; a second child in college might have strained his father's financial resources. In the fall of 1818, therefore, Edward was apprenticed to a woolen manufacturer in Stow. The experience proved a disaster. He was constantly at odds with his employer. Nor were his relationships with the other employees harmonious. They preferred to talk during their free moments, while Edward preferred to read, since he found their conversations ignorant and prejudiced.[10] Whether the difficulty in Stow was due to actual conditions or to Edward's resentment of his father and the frustration of his desire to attend college remains an enigma. Whatever the situation, Edward's rebellious behavior indicated that beneath the obedience he manifested in his parents' house lay strong emotions.

While in Stow, Edward became friendly with the Reverend Abraham Randall, a retired clergyman, who gave him access to his large personal library. Randall urged Francis Jarvis to send Edward to college, an opinion shared by Ripley. Following a final break with his employer, Edward returned home in the fall of 1820 and began to prepare for the entrance examinations to Harvard College. In early 1822 he began to teach school in Concord following the unexpected resignation of the regular instructor, thereby lessening the impending financial burden on his parents. The prospect of entering college acted as a stimulant; never had Edward worked so diligently at his studies. With the exception of Greek grammar, he passed the entrance examinations and entered Harvard College in the fall of 1822.[11]

By the early nineteenth century Harvard had abandoned its orthodox beginnings and become a center of liberalism and Unitarianism. Its most distinguishing feature during the first four decades of the nineteenth century was the dominant role played by a Unitarian faculty dedicated to what was then known as moral philosophy. Loosely defined, moral philosophy encompassed the study of human nature, metaphysics, and religion (especially natural theology). Indeed, moral philosophy served the same integrating and synthesizing function in antebellum American colleges as theology did in medieval universities. No Harvard student could have graduated without being exposed to the basic precepts of moral philosophy. Young Jarvis was surely no exception. If moral philosophy did not shape his perception of the world, it certainly confirmed his earlier training at home as well as in his church and school.

Moral philosophy was largely an outgrowth of eighteenth-century Scottish Common Sense philosophy, which was first formulated by Thomas Reid and further developed by others. Reacting against Hume's demonstration that the assumptions of Lockean empiricism could lead straight to a devastating skepticism, Reid was determined to restore belief in a knowable and objective external world. He began with the familiar argument that observation was the basis of knowledge, but then went on to assert that the mind contained innate principles that imposed order on the facts of experience. God, Scottish philosophers maintained, implanted common sense into the human mind, thereby enabling men to trust their senses and understand nature.

The victory of Unitarianism over Calvinism at Harvard at the beginning of the nineteenth century provided its faculty with an institutional base from which to develop moral philosophy and firmly implant its principles in the minds of several generations of students. The universe, moral philosophers insisted, was harmonious and orderly, and human beings possessed the capacity to understand its workings. Common sense realism sanctioned rational activity and restored confidence in both natural science and natural theology. Understandably, moral philosophy was especially compatible with the inductive and empirical method of Baconian science; the human mind was capable of observing the external world and deriving general laws from particular facts. Common sense, moreover, demonstrated that freedom of the will was a reality rather than an illusion; no further proof of its existence was required.

From such a philosophical perspective Harvard Unitarians could spell out a coherent ideology. They were firm believers in the perfectibility of man and insisted upon the paramount importance of the environment in molding character. Happiness and virtue were both achieved by the volitional acts of free human beings whose behavior conformed to the laws of nature. Rejecting irreconcilable class and social conflict, they posited the idea of an integrated and harmonious society under the leadership of a moral and educated elite. Moral philosophy, moreover, eliminated any incompatibility between science and religion; it endowed the former with the prestige of the latter, since the function of science was to collect the facts that would lead unerringly to a knowledge of the laws governing the universe.

Within this intellectual synthesis, education—broadly conceived—played a vital role. Education was both a religious and a moral imperative, for an orderly and harmonious society required a virtuous citizenry. Moral and regenerate individuals, by definition, were incapable of evil. Education was therefore the mediating force between the individual and society; ideally, self-realization was compatible with social harmony and order. Such views, of course, were well received in a society embarking upon rapid economic and technological development. It assured continued material progress while in no way undermining the position of dominant social and economic groups.[12]

Jarvis's four years at Harvard College were generally happy ones, as his subsequent concern with the fate of his alma mater demonstrated. Like other young men, he did not always take college as seriously as he could have; at the end of his first semester he was mortified to learn that he ranked fifty-sixth in a class of seventy-five. Determined to work harder, he increased his class standing and by the end of the second semester was ranked twenty-first. During his four years at Harvard he remained near the median; he gave no evidence of being an outstanding student.[13]

In the 1820s the Harvard curriculum was conventional. In the freshman year students studied Greek and Latin classics, algebra, geometry, and English grammar. In subsequent years they were introduced to analytic geometry and calculus, history, rhetoric, moral philosophy, political economy, and the sciences.

Jarvis was especially interested in botany, a fact that may very well have influenced his subsequent fascination with the classification of social phenomena. During the eighteenth century Linnaeus had all but erected the required framework of rules for taxonomy—the science of classification—and during the first half of the nineteenth century science was often defined in taxonomical terms. The Unitarian outlook that gave Harvard its character was completely compatible with taxonomy, for both presumed an orderly and meaningful universe. Indeed, in the decade following his graduation from college Jarvis continued to show considerable interest in botanical subjects,[14] a reflection of the fact that he felt most comfortable with concrete rather than abstract problems.

During three of the four winters he was a student at Harvard, Jarvis taught school, first in Acton, then in East Sudbury, and finally in Beverly. He did not find teaching an especially rewarding occupation, for his relationships with students left something to be desired. Yet the income relieved part of the burden on his father. The cost of Edward's education amounted to nearly $1,200 for four years, including $722 for tuition. Of this he earned $138 by teaching winters; the rest was provided by his father.[15]

In his senior year tragedy struck the Jarvis household. Edward's older brother Charles, with whom he was closest, became ill with a lung disease (probably tuberculosis). By October 1825 it began to dawn on the family that Charles would not recover. When Charles expressed the hope that Edward would return to Concord, he immediately complied. For nearly four months he was Charles's constant companion, having extricated himself from his teaching commitment for that winter. During these months the two brothers grew even closer. Charles confided in Edward that he was deeply disturbed by the fact that he would be unable to pay the money he had borrowed in order to attend the Harvard Medical School. In this respect the brothers were kindred souls; their notions of morality were similar to those of their father. On February 23, 1826, Charles passed away, leaving a void in Edward's life that was not easily filled.[16] Indeed, his brother's tragic death may very well have influenced Edward's subsequent decision to become a physician; before that he had given no indication whatsoever that the subject of medicine interested him.

Following Charles's death, Edward returned to Harvard. He had neglected his studies for more than four months. President John Kirkland, however, proved cordial and understanding; within a day he readmitted Jarvis with the sole proviso that he make up his lost studies. In April tragedy struck again when his mother, who had been ill with consumption for nearly a decade, also died. After her funeral Jarvis returned once again to Concord. On July 28 he left his beloved college for the last time as an undergraduate.[17]

III

Like other members of the Harvard Class of 1826 Jarvis desired success as well as the material rewards that followed. But—more importantly—he craved recognition from his fellow men. Indeed, during his brother's final ordeal he had a strange dream, which began with his own death and ascension to heaven. There Jarvis found a clear and light atmosphere with a soft haze, but without direct sunlight. Everywhere there were groups of cheerful people, all of whom knew and greeted him in a kindly and affectionate manner. At length he came to a group of four individuals who had been awaiting his arrival, for he was to be their associate. The group included William Ellery Channing, George Washington, Lord Chatham, and Thomas Aquinas. That Jarvis wished to be associated with such personalities was not surprising; throughout his adult career he always sought acceptance from renowned and distinguished figures. The four individuals of whom he dreamt also embodied many of the qualities that he most prized. All humanity recognized the feats of these men.[18]

Jarvis's hunger for recognition was but one facet of his now mature personality. By the time he attained his majority his character had taken its permanent form; he would show but few deviations from his basic behavioral patterns for the remainder of his long career. Among his most characteristic traits was a certain rigidity, which may have very well concealed feelings of insecurity or inferiority. He tended to see the world in terms of his own standards and predilections and was unable to concede any possibility of his own fallibility. His failures—if one is justified in even using that designation—were not the result of his own defects, but rather of the actions of others. Unable to accept differences, he insisted that the world accommodate itself to him; he lacked the flexibility that would have enabled him to operate on a more pragmatic level with others. Humanity, he averred, had an obligation to live up to a moral code given by a Divine Creator; no individual had a right to neglect duties and responsibilities or even to fulfill them in an imperfect or incomplete manner.

Along with his rigidity went a certain compulsiveness. Orderly to the extreme in his own behavior, Jarvis could not countenance disorder in the actions of others. Irregularity was an insult to nature's plan and bordered on the immorality that he so deeply abhorred. Every individual, whether child or adult, had an obligation to meet their responsibilities faithfully, and human frailty was no excuse. Consequently, Jarvis devoted as much time to minute details as he did to major problems.

Jarvis's relationships with others reflected his own rigid nature. He had relatively few close friends; those individuals with whom he claimed to be on intimate terms generally lived at a considerable distance and contacts with them were limited to exchanges of correspondence. His seeming inability to work with others was most vividly demonstrated in his failure to secure a position that would involve him with people. On the other hand, he functioned extraordinarily well with tasks that could be performed in isolation. Indeed, his career was marked by sheer intensity, productivity, and concentration; nothing that he undertook was performed in a haphazard manner.[19]

IV

At Harvard College Jarvis had received a superior education. The classical curriculum, however, had not prepared him for a career. Like other young college graduates, he began to ponder his future. His personal situation merely heightened the necessity of making a choice and becoming self-supporting. He could not rely upon his father and, unlike his eldest brother, was disinterested in the family business. A few months after his commencement in July 1826, moreover, Edward became engaged to Almira Hunt, daughter of a prosperous Concord farmer. His father reluctantly gave his consent, even though he thought the action precipitous because his son had no means of support. The announcement of the impending betrothal caused no surprise in this closely knit community.

Only six months younger than Jarvis, Almira Hunt proved an admirable choice as a partner. Intelligent and well-educated, she had taught school since the age of eighteen with considerable success. Devoted to Jarvis, she was capable of giving him the attention that he seemed to require. Although their marriage would not take place until 1834, the young couple grew closer together. Indeed, when Jarvis told his future bride about his diary and she apparently expressed some surprise, he wrote, "I am very sorry I did not tell her before. I have disclosed all my secrets (except this) to her & she has reciprocated the confidence. I will not be reserved on any other thing to her."[20]

In September 1826 Jarvis began to teach school in Concord. Finding little personal or financial satisfaction in teaching,[21] he began to consider other career alternatives. He was immediately attracted to the ministry, perhaps because of his strong attachment to Dr. Ripley. "The nature of the employment," he recalled in later years, "as teacher of holiness and as messenger from God to men, the opportunity to put forth those exact and devoted notions of right and wrong, of leading people, by love, to the paths of wisdom;—there seemed to him a beauty and a grace to this position and relation more than any other, and he wanted to devote his life and power to it." Jarvis's preference for the ministry was by no means unique; between 1636 and 1878 no fewer than 31 out of 108 college graduates from Concord became ministers. His friends, however, discouraged him from pursuing this profession, as had his brother Charles earlier. His speech was indistinct, and his enunciation imperfect, creating a serious impediment. Jarvis himself felt that he might also repel people, a fact that he attributed to his own severe notions of life and duty. Despite its overwhelming attractions, he decided against the ministry.[22]

Although law was the second most popular profession among Concord college graduates, Jarvis rejected this possibility. Instead he turned to medicine, though not without considerable misgivings. He did not object to the difficult preparation required, nor did he find the subject dry or uninteresting. Nevertheless, the profession brought practitioners into constant contact with disease, pain, and misery. Above all, the society of physicians was not of such quality as to offer sufficient inducement for an educated and cultivated mind. Indeed, physicians as a group, he noted, included in their ranks far less talent than other professions and had a far higher proportion of quacks. Medicine was decidedly not a literary profession; few physicians were interested in theory. For one who desired recognition and fame, a career as a physician seemed inappropriate. In spite of very real reservations, Jarvis, with some misgivings, decided to undertake the study of medicine.[23]

Jarvis's ambiguity toward medicine was not without a factual basis. The profession lacked a coherent structure; even states with licensing laws did not prohibit unlicensed practitioners. The training provided in medical schools did little to enhance the profession's standing; few institutions had minimum standards of admission, a graduated curriculum, or requirements for clinical experience. Some medical schools were created by enterprising entrepreneurs seeking rapid financial success. Many practicing physicians, moreover, never attended any school, but learned their trade through apprenticeship. The ambiguous status of the profession, however, was not due solely to structural weaknesses. Equally significant were internal divisions over appropriate modes of therapy; competing groups each proclaimed the superiority of their therapeutics. To many Americans the profession's inability to provide agreement on broad fundamentals was evidence of its failure; of all the sciences medicine was the least exact and the most backward.[24]

The seeming disarray within the medical profession, however, was partially balanced by the prestigious position of selected practitioners within specific communities. The decline of deferential personal relationships evident by the early nineteenth century weakened an important mechanism of social stability. The result was a corresponding increase in the importance of the traditional professions of law, medicine, and religion. Members of these professions increasingly assumed new social roles that transcended their immediate occupational responsibilities; they conceived of themselves as guardians and promoters of the general welfare. One byproduct was an elevation of the status of lawyers, clergymen, and physicians, particularly those concerned with more than routine performance of their duties. In Boston, for example, Drs. James Jackson and John C. Warren were closely associated with local elites in a variety of benevolent projects, including the founding of the Massachusetts General Hospital. Their careers (matched by comparable figures in other communities) demonstrated that physicians could attain considerable community eminence, particularly when medicine was defined in terms of the public welfare. In this sense Jarvis's decision to become a physician was compatible with his original desire to enter the ministry.

While teaching in Concord, Jarvis became an apprentice in the office of Dr. Josiah Bartlett, who dominated medical practice in that town until his death in 1878.[25] While fond of Bartlett, Jarvis made little progress in his medical studies. Teaching and community involvement left him little time for serious study. He also found that an apprenticeship in a physician's office was not synonymous with supervision or evaluation. Jarvis therefore decided that his interests and career would be better served by attending the Harvard Medical School and earning a degree. Such a move had financial implications. Jarvis might have borrowed money from his father; certainly the latter was in a position to raise the required funds even if his assets were not in liquid form. For some unknown reason Jarvis did not turn to his father. Instead, he accepted a loan from Samuel Hoar (one of Concord's best-known residents) sufficiently large to cover his expenses for about eighteen months. On October 15, 1827, Jarvis set off for Boston and two days later commenced his medical studies.[26]

Founded in 1782, the Harvard Medical School had a precarious existence during its early years. The high esteem it attained by the early nineteenth century was due less to the quality of its students or the nature of the instruction than to the distinction and high social status of its faculty, which enabled the institution to preserve its hold on medical education in the state. Instruction at the Harvard Medical School, on the other hand, left something to be desired. The education of young men was often limited to lectures, textbooks, and, to a lesser extent, the laboratory. The Massachusetts General Hospital, which was supposed to provide practical clinical experience, was far too small to accommodate the student body; before 1847 it never had more than seventy-two patients at one time. Students simply attended the lectures or clinical demonstrations, for which they purchased tickets, thereby providing the faculty with their source of income. The popular sentiment against dissection of human subjects made it difficult to secure bodies; not until 1830 did the Massachusetts legislature begin the process of legalizing anatomical dissection. The final examination administered to degree candidates rarely posed any serious impediments.[27]

At the Harvard Medical School Jarvis threw himself into his studies with characteristic intensity. During his first year he did not miss a single class. Instead of taking brief notes, he attempted to reproduce the lectures in verbatim form. The course of study was traditional: Jackson covered the theory and practice of medicine; Warren, anatomy and surgery; John Gorham, chemistry; Jacob Bigelow, the materia medica; and Walter Channing, midwifery and medical jurisprudence. In his three years in Boston, Jarvis found Jackson to be by far the most interesting and informative lecturer and regretted that his course lasted only three months. His attitude toward the others was more ambiguous.[28]

By the late 1820s the Harvard faculty was at a point midway between the older rationalistic medical systems with their generalized pathology and the newer French emphasis on detailed statistical investigations, a localized pathology, and a modified therapeutic nihilism. Within a few years, of course, French medicine dominated Harvard, as Jacob Bigelow's classic address in 1835 on the self-limited nature of disease demonstrated.[29] During Jarvis's stay in Boston, there was as yet little innovation. Jackson was already skeptical about traditional therapeutics, but he had not yet discovered Pierre Louis, whose statistical studies beginning in the mid-twenties had begun to undermine accepted forms of medical intervention. Consequently, Jackson retained many of the older practices. Nevertheless, his prescriptions tended to be milder than those of his colleagues, and he insisted that the function of the physician was to make the patient comfortable and avoid undue interference with natural processes.[30]

In conjunction with their courses, students were required to attend clinical sessions at the hospital, where they presumably viewed patients, studied diseases firsthand, and observed the influence of various therapeutic agents. Jarvis was dissatisfied with these visits. "I felt little interest in the cases," he wrote in his diary. "I knew nothing of practice, & the crowd in the wards prevented my having ready access to the patients." His comments were by no means unusual, for other students found their clinical experiences equally frustrating. Moreover, Jarvis found anatomy "abominably dull." In a characteristically extreme reaction he began to read widely in history, literature, and philosophy.[31]

Toward the end of June 1828 Jarvis was given an opportunity to accompany Dr. Benjamin Lincoln to Burlington, Vermont. Lincoln had accepted an appointment at the university to offer instruction in anatomy, surgery, and physiology. A rising figure in the medical profession, he had been friendly with Edward's recently deceased brother. Having received his M.D. degree only a year before, Lincoln hoped to compensate for his own relative inexperience in teaching by having a young medical student familiar with anatomical demonstration as his assistant; he asked Jarvis to accompany him to Vermont for three months. Jarvis would do all of the dissecting; in turn Lincoln would share with him his own extensive knowledge about anatomy and physiology.[32]

Lincoln's offer caused Jarvis some anxiety. He knew that the difficulty of securing corpses in Boston might deprive him of the opportunity of gaining vital dissection experience. On the other hand, he was not enthusiastic at the thought of leaving Boston. Several friends whose advice he solicited urged him to accept the offer. Jarvis finally agreed to go, although not before accepting his father's advice and rejecting Lincoln's generous offer of free lodgings and board.[33]

In late August Jarvis left Boston and visited Montreal before arriving in Burlington. Shortly thereafter Lincoln set him to work securing bodies and skeletons for instructional purposes. Jarvis demonstrated little moral anxiety over engaging in illegal activity; he may have convinced himself that the statutes forbidding anatomical dissection were wrong and could therefore be ignored. After some close brushes with law enforcement officials, Lincoln sent his young assistant on a trip south with instructions to procure human cadavers. During his three-week sojourn, Jarvis visited New York, Philadelphia, Baltimore, and Washington. In the former two cities he failed in his efforts, but in Baltimore he was able to strike a bargain with "the resurrection man" and purchase two bodies. These he packed in barrels, which accompanied him both on the stagecoach and aboard a ship on the way back. During these weeks Jarvis also met a number of prominent physicians and was able to observe life elsewhere. He was particularly disheartened after seeing slaves in the nation's capital. Slaves, he observed, are a "lazy, idle unprofitable race, doing not half the work a white can do . . . caring nothing for their owners interest. It would be a blessing to this country to transport the whole to Africa."[34]

After completing his stay in Vermont, Jarvis returned to Boston to continue his studies. The basic requirements for the M.D. degree at Harvard included attendance at two series of lectures (lasting approximately three to four months each), a three-year apprenticeship under a "regular practitioner of medicine," a dissertation upon some medical subject, and a final examination. Jarvis promptly became an apprentice at the office of George C. Shattuck, a Dartmouth graduate who entered practice in 1807. Shattuck's success drew students and patients alike to his office; Jarvis reported that he had been told that Shattuck carried the names of 4,000 patients on his books and earned at least $8,000 per year, a large sum for that period.[35]

Jarvis's apprenticeship experiences, however, were not especially rewarding. Indeed, a pattern quickly emerged that would be repeated on many future occasions. Whenever he worked in close proximity with others, friction would invariably follow.

Jarvis then would often rationalize the conflict in terms of the shortcomings of others. Consequently, he attributed his unhappy apprenticeship to Shattuck's conduct.[36]

Jarvis conceded that Shattuck would occasionally talk about his practice or give the names of diseases, but he rarely analyzed the history of an illness or the course of treatment. Indeed, instruction in his office was at best nominal. Although he was polite to his apprentices, he was sometimes "harsh, violent, & even rude to the poor, the weak, the ignorant, from whom he has no loss of good will." Shattuck's approach, insisted Jarvis, was to combat symptoms as they arose; he prescribed large quantities of medication, often after only a brief and cursory examination of the patient. His medical library was extensive, but most of the books had been published before 1818. Yet Jarvis had no ready explanation to account adequately for Shattuck's success other than to attribute it to a warm and affectionate bedside manner that inspired confidence and hope among patients.[37]

While working in Shattuck's office, Jarvis became deeply involved in a nearby dispensary located in an area with a large black and poor white population. He found the physician in charge to be a better and more sympathetic teacher than Shattuck. Between Shattuck's office and the dispensary, Jarvis saw large numbers of patients; he estimated that in the summer of 1829 alone he examined some three hundred persons. Charity patients were normally seen by the apprentices, although Shattuck was always willing to provide aid. For the first time in his life Jarvis came into contact with the Irish and other "low people, poor & dissolute." Somewhat insensitive to the feelings of others, he reported that these persons seemed to give him their full confidence. Yet, he noted in contradictory terms, they generally were "not very grateful. They like the doctor while he is healing them but . . . care nothing for him." Although his experiences in working with such patients proved instructive, Jarvis was not overly sanguine about the efficacy of treatment. It was fortunate that most diseases, if left alone, would disappear. The human constitution, he later recalled, would "bear not only much disease and interference, but also much disorder and medicine at the same time; consequently most of these poor patients recovered from their ailments when under the varied methods of treatment by these students.''[38]

During his stay in Boston Jarvis continued to see Almira as often as he could; rarely did a week pass without one or more visits with her. The years of waiting seemed to grow more oppressive; he could hardly wait to achieve the financial independence that would make their union a reality. The frequent visits to Concord also enabled Jarvis to become active in the town's affairs. He lectured before the Lyceum and in 1828 (together with Almira) joined Ripley's church, but not until the minister acceded to his refusal to make a public confession and accepted instead a simple statement about his belief in God, Christ, and the Bible, and a promise to live according to the precepts of Christianity.[39]

In the late summer of 1829 Jarvis was nearing the end of his medical studies. Upon Shattuck's advice he took a brief trip through central and western Massachusetts to observe medical practice outside of Boston. Following his return he resumed his apprenticeship in Shattuck's office and began to write his dissertation and prepare for his final examination.[40] Originally Jarvis had intended to prepare something that dealt with liver disorders, but he soon found this subject too vague and indeterminate. He finally decided to write on puerperal fever, partly because he could not find an easier or more appropriate topic. Two months later he completed a fifteen-page dissertation, which was shortly thereafter accepted by Channing. While several friends thought the paper of superior quality, there was little in it that deviated from conventional views of the subject.[41]

With his dissertation accepted and his apprenticeship completed, Jarvis was ready for his final examination. The month of January was devoted to an intensive review. It was common for students to conduct mock examinations in order to prepare for the ordeal. Jarvis took an active part in these preliminaries but, unlike some of his colleagues, did not show much anxiety about the outcome. Beneath the surface, however, may have lurked a feeling of insecurity; some months earlier he had questioned his ability to pass the examination. On the morning of January 26, Jarvis appeared before a faculty committee composed of Jackson, Warren, Webster, Channing, and Bigelow. No doubt Jarvis's confidence was strengthened by the knowledge that few students ever failed. The examination lasted between twenty-five and thirty minutes, and the committee then declared that Jarvis had passed. On February 2, Jarvis gave his dissertation a public reading; only Channing asked any questions. Two days later he received his diploma.[42] At the age of twenty-seven Jarvis had at last completed his education; his career was about to begin.

2

Frustration and Failure

A medical career in the 1830s was not—as it was to become a century later—a road to financial success. The profession seemed in a state of disarray, and its members were often unpopular because of widespread distrust of conventional therapeutics. Regular practitioners faced sharp challenges from sectarian groups who rebelled against traditional medical practice and substituted their own systems. The relative ease with which an individual could become a physician and the failure of attempts to institute a viable system of control through licensing often led to fierce competition. To be sure, a select group of physicians, by virtue of their contributions to the community, attained a position within the social structure that brought them status and affluence. The majority of practitioners, however, faced an environment certain to test their mettle.

For an individual with Jarvis's personality the going at best would be difficult. Faith in his superiority as a physician, when combined with a relative inflexibility, created problems. For slightly more than a decade he would find success and recognition beyond his grasp. But out of his failure would come a new career in the 1840s that would finally bring him the fame and material success he so ardently desired.

I

During the winter of 1830 Jarvis began to search for an appropriate community in which to establish a practice. To open an office in Concord, his first choice, was unrealistic. The town already had three physicians, and one of them—Josiah Bartlett—monopolized the affection and esteem of its citizens and was not enthusiastic about a new rival. Forced to consider other alternatives, Jarvis visited a number of communities in New Hampshire and Maine in early March, but none seemed attractive. Indeed, he may have rationalized his unwillingness to settle there by finding fault with the local townspeople.[1]

Upon his return to Concord, Jarvis was presented with an opportunity to open an office in Northfield, a small agricultural community some ninety miles northwest of Boston. The situation was made all the more attractive by the fact that his former classmate and friend George W. Hosmer had agreed to become the minister of the local church. Following a visit there, Jarvis decided to purchase a practice for two hundred dollars, and by the beginning of June had commenced his new career. The townspeople received him with cordiality and politeness, and his first impressions of them were equally favorable.[2]

Jarvis's initial venture into private practice was to prove less than successful. Indeed, a pattern quickly developed that was to be repeated on two more occasions between 1830 and 1842. Jarvis would move into a new community with hope and confidence; he would immediately attempt to integrate himself into its social, educational, and religious life. His enthusiasm, however, would prove short-lived, particularly when it became evident that his expectations for success were to prove unrealistic. His response was characteristic; he would immediately place responsibility for his failures upon the community.

For professional as well as personal reasons, Jarvis was disappointed with his situation. During his first six months in Northfield he earned only $131.20, a sum insufficient to cover the cost of acquiring the practice. Jarvis felt deceived, for he had been led to believe that he would clear between seven and eleven hundred dollars annually. Much to his amazement, the physician who sold the practice remained in town and continued to see patients. In addition, a third physician already monopolized more than one-half of the community's patients. Given the fact that Northfield had slightly less than eighteen hundred residents, his future prospects were anything but bright.[3]

In spite of an uneasy feeling that he had erred in coming to

Northfield, Jarvis attempted to integrate himself into the life of the community. He became active in the local lyceum, served on the town school committee, and gave lectures on chemistry and botany. He was also elected superintendent of the Sunday School, and soon thereafter prepared a series of lectures for the teachers that sought to demonstrate that anatomical structure and physiological processes were a reflection of the wisdom, benevolence, and design of the Creator.[4]

Jarvis's involvement in community affairs, nevertheless, did not compensate for his unhappiness, and his loneliness was allayed only by an occasional visit to Concord and Boston. "I am not contented," he wrote to Benjamin Lincoln. "I want better society, & more associates." He found his fellow townspeople lacking in refinement and literary qualities, and the cultural isolation of Northfield only contributed to his restlessness. Convinced that his reputation as a physician was on the rise, he remained puzzled by the smallness of his practice. During 1831 he earned slightly more than six hundred dollars, a sum that still fell short of his expectations. Consequently, the substantial debts that he had incurred in medical school remained unpaid. Under these circumstances it was difficult to contemplate marriage.[5]

Jarvis's practice, moreover, provided few compensations for his personal distress. With the possible exception of surgery (which he felt required "less exertion of intellect than ordinary practice"), his faith in medicine, which had never been strong, was eroded by his practical experiences. Rejecting a career as a surgeon, he found himself faced with a serious dilemma: how could he practice medicine if he lacked faith in prevailing therapies? Not long after leaving medical school he expressed in anguished terms his unhappiness to his former teacher and friend, Benjamin Lincoln. "I daily have less & less faith in the power of medicine," he wrote. He used, for example, antimony in the treatment of fevers. Some patients died, while others recovered; nor was the outcome significantly different if he abstained from any intervention. Given these results, did antimony do anything more than delude the physician into believing in the efficacy of his therapeutics and quieting the patient? "I have grown very skeptical as to medicine," he confessed. "I almost daily find that, from habit, I give things, & when I ask myself *what good will they do?* I cannot tell."[6]

Further contributing to his unhappiness was his perception of existing professional rivalries. His two colleagues in Northfield were "active & unprincipled" men who did not hesitate "at falsehood & defamation of character" if they believed that these tactics would enable them to steal business from him. "Our profession is low: it is humiliating to confess, how much, that is vile in it," he wrote in May 1832. "I did not know it, till I became an active member & entered the rivalry of practice." Responsibility for his unhappiness and failure had to reside elsewhere; he was unable to accept responsibility for his lack of success. "I once thought," he remarked a month later, "that correct principles, elevation of character, and thorough education would ultimately prevail. I may yet be right. But the time of such success is not so near at hand as once I thought it. I think less favorably of the world than I once did. I find on trial more ignorance more gullibility, more action from sinister motives than I hoped."[7]

Since his practice afforded him considerable (though involuntary) leisure time, Jarvis devoted himself to a variety of intellectual pursuits. He threw himself into the study of botany; explored metaphysics, especially the role of the mind in sensation; read law and history; and continued his medical studies. In early 1832 he became interested in cholera, which was then beginning to spread to the United States from abroad. By May Jarvis learned of outbreaks of the disease in Vermont, and he already anticipated its appearance in Northfield. Unfamiliar with the disease, he called upon Lincoln for information relative to symptoms and treatment. Jarvis rejected the contagionist argument even though he conceded that people were rendered more susceptible by close contact. At the urgings of James Jackson, with whom he remained on friendly terms, Jarvis collected information on an epidemic that had swept through Warwick (a small community adjacent to Northfield) the previous summer.[8] The result was the publication of his first article in early 1833 in the *Medical Magazine,* a short-lived journal edited by Jackson.

Jarvis's contribution was a relatively straightforward report of information on a local cholera epidemic. Like most physicians, he rejected the contagionist position as fallacious. His agreements with his professional brethren, however, did not imply unwillingness to question conventional wisdom. On the contrary, he was perfectly capable of taking unpopular positions, particularly when they were justified by evidence. He questioned, for example, the effectiveness of prevailing therapies—a stance which was hardly calculated to win popularity among his fellow practitioners. Nor did Jarvis moralize about cholera and attribute it to licentiousness or willful violation of natural law. Lacking any innovative qualities, the article did demonstrate a willingness to deal with theory in the light of hard evidence. It also illuminated a growing skepticism with conventional medical practice. Nevertheless, Jarvis was not yet ready to redirect his energies toward goals that differed significantly from the profession at large.[9]

Self-improvement and writing were sources of satisfaction to Jarvis, but they could not compensate for his inability to succeed as a practitioner of medicine. More and more, therefore, he began to turn inward and reflect upon his life. "I fear much my failure in this point," he observed only a year and a half after moving to Northfield. His character was not what it should have been; he had neglected the qualities of tenderness and delicacy in favor of strength, truth, and justice. Consequently, his usefulness to man and God was less than it could have been. A few months later he became even more introspective. Aware of his rigidity, he questioned if his stark interpretation of duty was simply a form of personal selfishness. He confessed a secret bias for notoriety; he wanted, above all, recognition, a desire "which all my self discipline & moral power has not yet removed." Imploring divine aid in overcoming character deficiencies, Jarvis was nonetheless unwilling to accept sole responsibility for his failure. Northfield was "not the place" for an individual like himself. "My motive was to obtain immediate business & I did," he observed in words that belied reality. "But whenever business is immediately obtainable by a young man generally there are either few competitors, or they are worthless, & the place will not afford all that an ambitious man will hope to

deserve when he shall have gained knowledge by experience.
. . . I am not willing to continue thro my life as I now am. I am
determined to be a better physician & a greater & more useful
man each year as I advance in life.''[10]

II

At the end of September 1832 Jarvis decided to visit Concord,
since he had no patients requiring his presence. Upon his arrival
he was greeted with an astonishing piece of news. One of the active physicians in Concord had decided to leave, creating an
unparalleled opportunity. After consulting with his father, fian-
cée, and friends, Jarvis decided to make the move; by October
he was settled amidst familiar surroundings.[11]

Within weeks Jarvis's new environment had completely altered
his outlook and mood. Any doubts about his eventual success
disappeared. Whereas the people of Northfield neither understood nor appreciated him, the residents of Concord treated him
''with much confidence & Kindness'' both in professional and
in social and civil relations. The latter were far more intelligent
and less gullible; he would no longer have to contend with the
pernicious lies spread by unprincipled rivals. His newly found
happiness was tempered by a recognition that he had still done
''comparatively little.'' His dreams were dominated by feelings
of virtue, purity, and goodness, but these qualities remained
elusive and seemingly beyond his grasp. Why, Jarvis asked himself, should he search for them ''when it is so far from the actual
circumstances & means of my being.'' Such thoughts did not occupy his mind for long. ''I have no reason to regret my removal,'' he wrote to Lincoln, ''for the Concordites are not so
stiffnecked as the Jews of old, & will yield a prophet some
honour in his own country.''[12]

Initially the success that was so elusive in Northfield seemed
within reach in Concord. Each month his practice and income
increased. In view of brighter prospects, his marriage to Almira
Hunt took place on January 9, 1834. Still in debt, the newly-
weds lived as frugally as possible. Fortunately, financial prob-

lems did not lead to domestic friction. Strong in her own right, Almira was able to provide her husband with affection and security. Nor did the absence of children impair the development of a happy and satisfying relationship.[13]

To Jarvis, Concord was more than his place of business; it was one of the most desirable communities in the country. As in Northfield, he immersed himself in a variety of community activities, none of which were inspired by a desire to expand his practice. He became active in Ripley's church, served on the town school committee, and was active in the Social Circle, a club that attempted to preserve the memories of eminent residents and sponsored discussions of all important questions of town policy. Similarly, Jarvis joined the Concord Lyceum, which had been founded in 1828 and quickly brought eminent speakers to the town. Shortly thereafter he became a curator and assumed responsibility for the management of its lecture series. In addition to administrative functions, he often gave lectures and engaged in debates. Invariably his presentations emphasized the indissoluble and organic ties that bound the moral, social, and scientific orders. One of his first lectures dealt with the freedom of the human mind; succeeding ones emphasized the immortality of the soul and harmony of the biological world. His basic concerns, however, were less with abstractions and more with specific and contemporary policy issues. On various occasions he argued for the innate intellectual superiority of whites as compared with blacks; he opposed immediate emancipation of slaves, while supporting antislavery agitation; he favored freedom of the press but feared indiscriminate reading of novels; he urged that representatives be bound by the instructions of their constituents; he thought the French Revolution more productive of evil than good; he favored the abolition of capital punishment; and he attempted to refute the belief that climate produced racial differences. To Jarvis the world could be understood only in moral categories; it was futile to attempt to separate either science or politics from the moral order. His own experiences with medicine and people simply strengthened his perception that egocentric and selfish behavior was responsible for the persistence of social problems. The function of the lyceum was no different from the function of public or religious schools; it provided a vehicle to educate citizens and direct them toward wisdom and goodness. [14]

Predictably, Jarvis maintained that contemporary problems were resolvable only by reference to general principles; he did not temper strongly held convictions with a sense of pragmatism or skepticism. In 1833, for example, he was angered when a fair was held in Boston for the purpose of raising money to aid the blind. In an article for the *New England Magazine* he charged that people were being compelled to spend their money because of the "influence of the benevolent sisterhood," which had acquired the power to grant or to withhold its approval without any restraint. If the goal was the support of philanthropy, why could not contributions be solicited directly? These fairs, moreover, encouraged undesirable behavioral traits by sanctioning gambling. The end did not justify the means, for "whatever principle is shown to be wrong, in the abstract, certainly no application, to however pure purpose, or in however virtuous hands, can justify its operation." [15]

III

Interestingly enough, Jarvis's immersion in Concord's social and public life was not matched by professional success. Indeed, after four years in Concord he was still unable to repay any of his debts; only by observing the most rigid economies was he able to remain self-supporting. His closest friends treated him with affection and kindness, but most of them engaged Bartlett as their physician. Perhaps Jarvis's personality repelled prospective patients. Perhaps his distrust of traditional medical practices did not stand him in good stead with people seeking definitive advice and optimistic treatment of their ills. Whatever the reasons, his anxieties and unhappiness grew more intense. Lacking insight into his own character, he was unable to adjust in ways that might have made others more comfortable in his presence. Responsibility for failure again had to be found outside of himself. [16]

Jarvis's disillusionment with medical intervention and his inability to build a successful practice strengthened his growing conviction that medical theories and practices were in error. But if the practice of medicine was a charade, what was the role of the physician? Convinced of the purity of his own motives, Jarvis was unable to explain his lack of success without seeing others in a negative light. Although he would not formulate comprehensive answers to the questions that troubled him for some years to come, it was evident that his Northfield and Concord experiences contributed to his growing receptivity for alternative approaches.

At about this time Jarvis became familiar with the quantitative approach that was already beginning to dominate European and particularly French medicine. The application of a statistical methodology, of course, was not of recent origin; the theory of mercantilism rested upon the belief that the quantitative data of natural life could result in knowledge that would enhance the authority and power of the nation-state. Such figures as William Petty (who coined the phrase political arithmetic) and John Graunt were acutely aware of the relationship between a healthy and growing population and national power; they emphasized the benefits that would accrue to policy officials from accurate knowledge of health-related problems. Indeed, the latter's most famous work in 1662 involved an analysis of mortality rates in London during the preceding third of a century. By the eighteenth century the possibilities inherent in a statistical analysis of disease were made more explicit by philosophers like Condorcet and physicians like Philippe Pinel. The philosophy of Ideology, with its empirical approach, markedly strengthened faith in analytic statistics.[17] Industrial and technological changes, which created new social problems, also reinforced interest in an approach that held out the possibility of developing policies that would prevent disease and thus increase productivity. Finally, the rise of the Paris school of medicine in the half century following 1800 proved of critical importance to the formulation of Jarvis's thought. Figures such as Bichat and others moved away from the generalized pathology so characteristic of rationalistic medicine and attempted instead to identify specific disease entities in terms of a localized and structural pathology. In this environment Pierre Louis undertook his numerical studies of disease by observing large numbers of ward cases and performing numerous post mortems. In 1835 he spelled out in detail the principles of his "numerical method" and thereby stimulated interest in applying a quantitative methodology to a variety of health-related problems. All of these developments raised serious doubts about the effectiveness of traditional therapeutic intervention.[18]

Intellectually and emotionally Jarvis was drawn to a view of medicine that seemed to resolve all of his inner doubts. His Unitarian upbringing and education in Common Sense philosophy already made him receptive to an approach that presupposed an orderly and rational universe. His training in taxonomical botany helped to shape his ability to classify facts in clear and objective categories; it was only a small step to move from classification to collection of aggregate data. A quantitative approach also appealed to him on personal grounds. It would prove beyond a reasonable doubt that the conventional practices of most physicians were useless or fraudulent. Statistics would eliminate all personal and subjective elements and force the profession to deal with facts whose validity was beyond doubt. To put it another way, the personal attributes of the physician would play no role in the determination of his competency or status; success would be based exclusively on objective criteria. In discrediting the basis of prevailing medical practice, Jarvis implicitly placed responsibility for his own lack of success as a physician elsewhere.

But a view of medicine that rested on a quantitative methodology appealed to Jarvis for other reasons as well. By illuminating the individual and social factors that caused disease, the physician would assume a critical role in society. He would provide both the essential information that had to precede the formulation of proper public and private policies and serve as a prophet and teacher by exposing current evils and offering definitive and authoritative statements of proper behavioral norms. Ideally, physicians would occupy the role reserved by Plato for philosophers; the only difference was that medicine rather than philosophy would wed knowledge and wisdom, and thereby aid mankind in the quest to establish a better world. The profession of medicine, therefore, differed little from the profession of religion; the role and functions of physicians and ministers were similar. "This seemed to be the true field of professional inquiry," Jarvis recalled,

> and in this way it seemed the physician should make himself useful to his fellows and hold himself ready as a prophylactic adviser to warn the people of danger and keep them in the path of health. So the world should look upon the medical profession, as guardians of their health, and consult its memories as to the management of their lives; as the commercial and financial world consult the legal profession, and obtain their guidance in the legal and sure way of administration of business and property.[19]

By the 1830s knowledge of European medical developments had been widely disseminated among a number of American physicians. As a medical student Jarvis had read Xavier Bichat, whose classic work on pathological anatomy rejected a nosology based on outward symptoms in favor of one that incorporated symptoms and lesions. Jarvis's continuing contact with Jackson after graduation from medical school may have introduced him to Pierre Louis, since Jackson emerged as an enthusiastic supporter of the statistical study of disease. It is certain that Jarvis read Louis' work shortly after its publication in France in 1835 and was immediately convinced that the numerical method was "the only true way."[20]

Whatever its origins, Jarvis's commitment to a quantitative approach to the study of disease matured following his return to Concord. His growing affinity for quantification was presaged by the publication of a paper dealing with intemperance and disease in the prestigious *Boston Medical and Surgical Journal* in 1836; this paper was based on data collected by Jarvis and Bartlett (both of whom feared intemperate drinking). Dissatisfied with mere moral exhortation, Jarvis used his collected data as the basis for an analysis of the relationship between alcoholism and disease. Unwilling to rest his case on moral grounds alone, he attempted to prove the validity of his warnings about the harmful effect of drinking. By dividing his patients into non-drinkers and temperate and intemperate drinkers, he was able to show that the first group had a lower incidence of sickness. From here it was but a short step to conclude that a causal relationship existed between alcohol and disease. Moreover, Jarvis provided additional data to demonstrate that intemperate patients defaulted upon their debts with a far greater frequency than did temperate drinkers or abstainers. "Even the most selfish of our profession," he concluded, "may join the temperance cause."[21]

Especially notable about Jarvis's article was the fact that he had begun with the belief that drinking was undesirable, and had then attempted to demonstrate that the evidence confirmed the thesis. Replete with figures, his essay was based upon simple cross tabulation. Convinced that alcohol was dangerous, he did not consider other variables. Classification and statistical analysis thus became in part the means of objectifying his own moral preconceptions.

While gathering materials on intemperance, Jarvis encountered his first case of mental illness. In the fall of 1835 a young man suffering from a mild case of insanity was brought to him, described as a "distressed monomaniac." His constant wailing caused his family considerable anxiety. Since his private practice was not large, Jarvis consented to take the individual into his home and provide proper care and treatment. By the following spring the patient had recovered sufficiently to return home. In due course two additional patients were referred, one of them by James Jackson. These cases turned Jarvis's attention to insanity, a subject that he quickly found "more consonant to his mental habits and taste than the care of physical disease."[22]

That Jarvis found the subject of insanity intriguing was not surprising. The fact that only a handful of physicians were interested in mental disease meant that opportunities awaited a young man seeking a career in a new specialty. Moreover, psychiatric practice at this time meant institutional practice; a hospital superintendency offered security and a measure of recognition, both of which had thus far eluded Jarvis. More importantly, the prevailing concepts of insanity were especially appealing to him, for they confirmed his faith in the orderly and moral nature of the universe.

The mid-nineteenth-century model of mental disease was a blend of ideas. It included sensationalist and associationist psychology, phrenology, and behaviorism, as well as ideas borrowed from Scottish Common Sense philosophy. Most psychiatrists be-

Frustration and Failure   41

gan with Lockean assumptions; they believed that knowledge came to the mind through sensory organs. If the senses (or the brain) became impaired or diseased, false impressions would be conveyed to the mind, leading in turn to faulty thinking and abnormal behavior. Phrenology, which gained a rapid foothold in America after being imported from Europe in the 1820s and 1830s, provided a means of connecting mind and matter. The mind, according to phrenological theorists, was not unitary, but was composed of independent and identifiable faculties, which were localized in different regions of the brain. To this theory phrenologists added the belief that individuals could deliberately and consciously cultivate different faculties by following the natural laws that governed physical development and human behavior. The popularity of phrenology seemed to confirm the psychiatric belief that all normal and abnormal functions of the mind were dependent on the physical condition of the brain.

Such reasoning provided psychiatrists with a medical model of mental illness that was especially compatible with a psychological and environmental etiology. Mankind, they reasoned, was governed by certain immutable natural laws that provided a guide to proper living. If these laws were violated, the physical organs (including the brain) would not develop or function normally. In other words, mental illness, though somatic in nature, could have psychological as well as physical causes. Thus it was the abnormal or immoral behavior of the individual (who possessed free will) that was the primary cause of insanity, leading as it did to the impairment of the brain. Mental illness, therefore, was in some cases self-inflicted; by ignoring (or being ignorant of) the laws governing human behavior, the individual placed himself on the road to disease.

From such beliefs psychiatrists drew the natural conclusion that mental illness was as curable as, if not more curable than, other somatic diseases. If derangements of the brain and nervous system produced the various types of insanity, it followed that the removal of such causal abnormalities would result in the disappearance of the symptoms and therefore the disease. Treatment fell into two broad categories: medical and moral (i.e., psychological). The former involved a range of traditional medicinal agents, including drugs, tonics, and laxatives. Medical treatment of insanity, however, was but a prelude to what in the nineteenth century was known as moral treatment. While susceptible to many interpretations, moral treatment meant kind, individualized care in a small institution with occupational therapy, religious observance, amusements and games, and in large measure a repudiation of physical violence and an infrequent resort to mechanical restraint. Moral treatment in effect involved re-educating the patient in a proper moral atmosphere.[23]

Such a theoretical model of disease appealed to Jarvis, partly because it seemed to confirm the validity of his personal belief in a moral universe where right and wrong were clearly delineated. In typical fashion he threw himself into the study of insanity and within four years had read virtually every significant work on the subject.[24] The notion that insanity was partially self-inflicted fitted with his growing conviction that the prophylactic and didactic functions of physicians took precedence over all others. His affinity for psychiatry was further strengthened by the prevailing etiological concept that mental illness often resulted either from individual immorality or a deficient social order that reflected acquisitive and competitive values. It was understandable that Jarvis, disillusioned by his experiences in private practice, would be drawn to a specialty that placed a large measure of responsibility for individual and social problems on a nation that had partially lost sight of its original values. "I wish to trace out Insanity to its sources," he later recalled when recounting his first involvment with mental illness, "in original organization, in development, in education, in habits of life, in customs of society, in the thousand trials & temptations that surround us. It seems to me, that much good may [be] done by this course, & the disease, in a great measure, be prevented in future generations."[25]

In late 1836 Jarvis was presented with an exceptional opportunity when the superintendency of the McLean Asylum for the Insane (a separate division of the Massachusetts General Hospital) became vacant upon the death of Dr. Thomas G. Lee. Opened some eighteen years earlier, McLean had become one of the nation's leading private hospitals. Jarvis's candidacy was presented to the trustees by James Jackson, and Emerson wrote a strong supporting letter emphasizing his "great energy & usefulness" to the people of Concord, "his industry, his love of system, & his public spirit." Jarvis was ecstatic at the prospect of securing a position that was admirably suited to his temperament and character. The annual salary of $1,500, plus quarters and board, also promised an end to his financial problems. The rival candidate was Dr. Luther V. Bell, who had come to prominence during a struggle in the New Hampshire legislature over passage of a law establishing a public mental hospital. Despite the support of Jackson and several trustees, Jarvis did not receive the position. Conceding that Bell was an excellent choice, he nevertheless attributed his failure to the decisive role played by the Reverend Louis Dwight, secretary of the influential Boston Prison Discipline Society. To Jarvis the decision came as a bitter blow. "O could I have gone there!," he wrote. "I wanted to go. I tried to go. I prayed God to grant me the place. But it was not determined that I should be then the physician of the McLean Asylum."[26]

While Jarvis was awaiting the decision of the McLean trustees, several of his friends who had travelled through Kentucky—including the Reverend George W. Hosmer—urged him to consider a move to Louisville, a rapidly growing city lacking trained physicians. In September James Freeman Clarke, the young liberal Unitarian minister who was instrumental in bringing Transcendentalism to the West, visited Concord and spoke in glowing terms of Louisville. During his stay he attempted to convince Jarvis to migrate to a region noted for its opportunities. So long as McLean remained a viable possibility, Jarvis avoided making a decision. Upon learning that he would not be offered the superintendency, he decided in a somewhat abrupt and impulsive manner to make the move. The prospect of leaving a familiar environment did not prove a deterrent. Still seeking the success that continued to elude his grasp, he determined to begin his career anew.[27]

IV

On March 2, 1837, Jarvis left Concord for Boston. The following day he went to Providence and boarded a boat for New

York. His first long stop was in Philadelphia, where he spent nearly a week speaking with prominent physicians, soliciting letters of recommendation, and observing medical facilities and, perhaps for the first time, welfare institutions. Jarvis was impressed with the local medical profession, partly because many of its members shared his own distrust of medication and were willing to "believe the agency of nature in recovery of her own ills." He found the Pennsylvania Hospital to be under excellent management, but was appalled by conditions in the almshouse. Reflecting the prevailing antebellum belief that pressing social problems could be resolved by molding and reshaping the character of individuals, he did not dissent from the proposition that institutions had vital roles to play in American society. Whether speaking about the virtues of mental hospitals, schools, or penitentiaries, Jarvis, like other activists of his generation, held out the hope that crime, disease, and dependency could eventually be eradicated by these structures. His favorable reaction to the penitentiary, an institution already well known for its rehabilitative activities, was typical. The basic problem of prisons, he noted in his journal, was that they tended to mix diverse people in an indiscriminate manner. Ideally, hardened criminals should be separated from other inmates, some of whom had stolen simply to ensure the survival of their families. Jarvis favored indeterminate rather than fixed sentences; punishment ought to be evaluated "solely by its effects, & this be a cure of the moral disease."[28]

From Philadelphia Jarvis proceeded to Lancaster and Harrisburg, and then to Pittsburgh. After spending several pleasant days in Marietta, Ohio, he arrived in Cincinnati and quickly sought out Dr. Daniel Drake, a figure already famous for his leadership in medical education and studies of various diseases. The city's medical profession, however, was not favorably disposed toward Pierre Louis' method of analysis, and Jarvis quickly found himself cast in the role of defender. By this time his outlook was more confident and optimistic; he was certain that Providence would guide him toward his predestined goals.[29]

On April 18 Jarvis resumed his travels and two days later arrived in Louisville. His first impressions were not favorable.

Lacking architectural elegance, the city was dominated by a variety of commercial enterprises. Perhaps more than anything else, Jarvis was struck by the presence of slave and free blacks. Although hostile toward the institution of slavery, his attitude toward blacks was ambivalent; he found their moral character lacking in important respects. On the other hand, Jarvis conceded, involuntary servitude militated against the development of the physical and moral senses, a fact recognized by all. He was equally unimpressed with the local residents, whose drinking and profanity offended him. He may have mentally compared Louisville with Concord and found the former deficient in most respects.[30]

The city to which Jarvis had migrated was relatively young. Founded just after the American Revolution, Louisville experienced slow growth before 1800. Its strategic location at the falls of the Ohio River, however, made it a key port for transportation and communication between New Orleans and the developing Midwest. The advent of the steamboat sealed the city's future; its development as a manufacturing and mercantile center was assured. Between 1820 and 1840 the population increased from 4,000 to 21,000. Such rapid growth provided physicians with innumerable opportunities, especially since the large ponds of stagnant water located in adjacent low areas gave the town the unenviable reputation as the graveyard of the West. Although conditions had improved by 1837, there was little doubt that the community was attractive to young practitioners about to launch a career.[31]

Upon his arrival Jarvis set up an office in the business district not far from the waterfront. Hitherto a relatively stable neighborhood, this district was hard hit by the depression that began in 1837; within two years there were no fewer than thirty-two changes of occupants in nineteen establishments. Nevertheless, the severe economic decline did not inhibit people from employing physicians, and much to Jarvis's delight his practice thrived from the outset. During his first full year his billings totalled $2,960; in the succeeding two years his practice levelled off at about $2,400 each year. His expenses were modest, averaging slightly over one thousand dollars per annum. Under these circumstances financial success seemed assured.[32]

The patients who consulted Jarvis in Louisville did not differ from those he had seen in the past. Indeed, he was surprised that diseases in Louisville were similar to those in Massachusetts. Jarvis's skepticism, however, was by this time too deeply embedded to permit him to accept prevailing diagnoses or therapeutics. "Bilious seems to be the universal name for disease and calomel the universal remedy," he wrote in caustic terms to Jackson. "Families keep their bottle of calomel as commonly as they keep oil or salts in their houses in New England." His sarcastic tone to the contrary, there is little evidence that Jarvis employed unorthodox forms of medical intervention.[33]

When Jarvis arrived in Louisville, the medical profession in the city and state was engaged in fratricidal warfare. Rivalries between the faculty of the Medical Department of Transylvania University in Lexington—by far the most eminent of the western medical schools—and those unable to secure comparable appointments created pressure for new schools. Following a bitter and acrimonious conflict betwen Lexington and Louisville, the Louisville Medical Institute commenced operations in the fall of 1837. Within a few years the new faculty had attracted a number of distinguished figures, including Dr. Daniel Drake and Dr. Samuel D. Gross.[34]

In Louisville the establishment of the Medical Institute aroused sharp antagonisms between the faculty and local physicians seeking similar appointments in order to enhance their reputation and hence increase their practice. Convinced that both sides were partly to blame, Jarvis attempted to follow a course midway between both extremes and thereby retain the friendship and respect of all. There was little doubt that during his stay in Louisville he was unhappy with the fragmented state of the profession. If medicine was to serve as the teacher of humanity, how could its followers continue to fight among themselves in ways that threw the profession into disrepute? No doubt he agreed with the judgment of an old friend and colleague that "the West is not what it is 'cracked up to be.' . . . The society falls far short of our Eastern notwithstanding what it thinks of itself. And the profession in the West is a perfect waste, made up of all discordant elements, quackery & nostrum."[35]

V

Jarvis's negative reaction to Louisville was not accompanied by a refusal to participate in its public or religious life. On the contrary, he hoped to impose the superior morality and customs of Massachusetts upon his adopted state and thus elevate the character of its people. His didactic and prophylactic view of medicine only strengthened his conviction that he could not remain aloof or isolated. From the very moment of his arrival he became an active participant in community affairs, thus repeating the pattern he had established first in Northfield and then in Concord.

Much to Jarvis's satisfaction, Louisville had a young and vigorous Unitarian Church whose minister, James Freeman Clarke, was a fellow New Englander. A resident of the city from 1833 to 1840, Clarke also edited the *Western Messenger,* which printed contributions by leading Transcendental authors. In Clarke Jarvis found a kindred spirit, since both men linked religion with spiritual and material progress, and neither was interested in abstract theological questions. So attractive was Clarke's Unitarianism that Jarvis within a two-year span found time to write three articles for the *Western Messenger* summarizing his personal views of God, humanity, and ethics.

The occasions of his first two articles in 1838 were a revulsion against the inhumane treatment of animals and the death of Nathaniel Bowditch. In both Jarvis dealt with the subjects in terms of general moral principles. Similarly, in his discussion of the New England Non-Resistance Society two years later Jarvis found room for disagreement while simultaneously upholding commitment to principle. In 1838 a group of pacifists dissatisfied with the American Peace Society formed the New England Non-Resistance Society and rejected absolutely the use of force under any circumstances (although agreeing to submit "to the penalty of disobedience"). Jarvis could not help but admire the small but resolute group of men and women; they were people who refused to forsake principle for expediency or personal gain.[36]

Moral exhortation was but one path to social enlightenment. Equally important was the dissemination of knowledge that would build character and develop the inner discipline and self-restraint that would enable individuals to resist temptation. To Jarvis Louisville and the West were in need of more institutionalized means to socialize and to channel behavior. In New England society was cemented by "pervading public opinions"; individuals were but parts of an organic whole. In the West, on the other hand, society was atomized into an "infinite variety of unassimilated elements." If an individual's religious character was well-developed, the West, precisely because of its emphasis on individualism and self-reliance, simply strengthened what already existed. But for those who required institutional support and checks and restraints characteristic of the organic social order of New England, the West was an inappropriate place. Indeed, those whose characters were defective should be discouraged from migrating; they required the "rigid social influence of New England" to restrain their behavior.[37]

To Jarvis formal schooling was destined to play an increasingly important role in educating and socializing the people of Louisville. In the summer of 1838 he therefore accepted an appointment to the Board of School Visitors, a position that he retained until the spring of 1842. In this capacity he devoted considerable time and energy to improving the quality of schooling and increasing the level of funding. As far as Jarvis was concerned, Louisville schools were distinctly inferior to Massachusetts schools. "We are a century behind you in education of the people," he wrote to Horace Mann. "A slaveholding state cannot appreciate an educated labourer as you do. Our city is doing much for its schools, and we hope to make them yet more profitable to our children, and by the aid of your counsel & your examples we may follow in the footsteps of Mass."[38]

In his official capacity as a visitor, Jarvis worked to impose the rationale and organization of the Massachusetts school system upon Louisville. Already acquainted with Mann, he disseminated the latter's influential reports among colleagues. His justification for education, like Mann's, was phrased in broad terms. Education contributed "to happiness and to virtue, to social and domestic comfort, to public order and to private profit . . . [O]ur government and our people should look after and cherish our common schools, if they wish to secure honor and prosperity to the State, if they wish to gain wealth and happiness, political and social advantage for themselves and their children.'' A proper system of universal free education could not but benefit the individual as well as society. For if disease, intemperance, premature mortality, an overdeveloped sense of acquisitiveness—to mention only a few conditions—were the result of character shortcomings, might not schools, by molding children during their formative years, help to eradicate defects and contribute toward the creation of a better world?[39]

During Jarvis's stay in Louisville the number of schools nearly tripled. Such rapid expansion, however, did not come without opposition. In 1842 the city council abolished the Board of School Visitors and created a new board. Some of the resentment toward the old agency arose because of the dominance of ''Yankees'' and their efforts to model Louisville after Boston. The council also wanted parents with sufficient resources to pay tuition. Opposition to the council surfaced almost immediately. Although stripped of his membership on the board and already contemplating his return to New England, Jarvis was gratified at the eventual victory of his supporters.[40]

VI

Although Jarvis had little or no opportunity to specialize in cases of insanity after leaving Concord, his interest in the subject never wavered. He continued to read extensively and to collect materials from American and foreign sources. Under ordinary circumstances the arduous demands of general practice might have left him with little spare time. But his initial success in Louisville proved of short duration. After his first year his real income began to decline, a pattern not unlike his previous experiences in Northfield and Concord. His inability to maintain a successful practice, therefore, left him with time to pursue other interests and made him receptive to the possibility of an alternative career pattern that promised to compensate for past failures.

A newly settled state, Kentucky nevertheless established the nation's second public mental hospital in 1824. In providing custodial rather than therapeutic care, the Eastern Lunatic Asylum in Lexington reflected few of the newer concepts of mental illness or the role of institutionalization for the first two decades of its existence.[41] Jarvis's discovery that the Kentucky Asylum bore little resemblance to Eastern institutions like McLean galvanized him to action. Here was an opportunity to put to good use his extensive knowledge of mental illness. The citizens of Kentucky had taken the first step when they had established a hospital two decades earlier. They had acted with the best of motives, but their actions were based on partial ignorance. What was now required was a careful analysis of all relevant data that would at once expose existing defects and illuminate the contours of future policy.

For more than three years Jarvis gathered materials on the care and treatment of the insane. One of the very first problems he faced was that of acquiring appropriate data. At that time there were no research libraries, and medical schools paid little or no attention to the systematic collection of scientific literature. Knowledge of significant medical findings often failed to be transmitted to a profession that lacked systematic means of disseminating information among its members. The problem in regard to mental illness was even more acute. A professional self-identity was still to be achieved; during the 1830s there were fewer than two dozen American physicians who might have admitted to being specialists on the subject. Aside from its intrinsic importance, the collection and analysis of data appealed to an individual with systematic work habits. Such work could be performed in isolation; Jarvis would not have to contend with other individuals. Finally, the results of his work could be presented in irrefutable factual and statistical form, thereby dispelling the errors and false opinions that hitherto had determined public policy.[42]

The first concrete result of Jarvis's labors was a short article in the *Boston Medical and Surgical Journal* that described the care of the insane in Kentucky.[43] This piece was but a prelude to two longer articles on mental illness that appeared initially in the *Western Journal of Medicine and Surgery* and then, owing largely to Jarvis's own efforts, circulated nationally in pamphlet form. The first was a review of recent psychiatric literature; the second a discussion of public policy toward insanity in the West.

Taken together, they presaged the beginnings of a new career for Jarvis. Ultimately this career would bring him recognition and a reputation as one of the most important American psychiatrists of the mid-nineteenth century, a figure who ranked with men like Isaac Ray, Pliny Earle, and Thomas S. Kirkbride.

The first article was ostensibly a review of W.A.F. Browne's lectures on insanity (published in 1837 in Edinburgh) and twenty-three annual reports of American mental hospitals. In reality, it was more a highly accurate summary of contemporary psychiatric thought and practice that demonstrated familiarity with such European and English figures as Pinel, Esquirol, Tuke, and Prichard, and Americans such as Earle, Brigham, Bell, and Woodward, to say nothing of investigations by state legislatures and foreign governments.

Accepting the prevailing faith that psychiatry had arrived of age and that mental disease could be cured, Jarvis briefly recounted the dismal history of past treatment of the insane. Beginning with Pinel in the 1790s, however, a new age had dawned. Hospitals now assumed a therapeutic rather than a custodial function; to demonstrate this fact Jarvis proceeded to describe virtually every public and private institution in the United States and many foreign ones as well. He emphasized the beneficial results of institutionalization, pointing to recovery rates of recent cases (defined as having been insane for one year or less) that ran as high as 90 percent or more. A beneficent and enlightened public policy was far more economical than a repressive one; the statistics graphically demonstrated that it was cheaper to cure people than to maintain them for long periods of time in welfare institutions.

As accurately as anyone else, Jarvis caught the confident and optimistic mood that was so characteristic of American psychiatry. Implied, but not yet spelled out in detail, was the assumption that the elimination of mental illness was within the grasp of the American people if only they showed the wisdom and foresight to make the necessary financial investment. Jarvis's only reservations related to the Kentucky Asylum, and he urged the legislature to launch an investigation and also offered a brief series of proposals designed to make the state a leader rather than a laggard in caring for its insane.[44]

In his second article three months later, Jarvis urged Westerners to establish a modern mental hospital, preferably near the Ohio or Mississippi Rivers so as to be easily accessible. Surely, he concluded, the five million inhabitants of the region possessed "intelligence enough to appreciate such an institution; benevolence enough to desire it, and wealth sufficient to create it and put it into successful operation."[45]

The initial reaction to Jarvis's appeal was gratifying. The Louisville *Daily Journal* urged legislative action. Similar commendation came from the *Boston Medical and Surgical Journal*, which reprinted a substantial portion of Jarvis's first article.[46] The response of the Kentucky legislature also seemed favorable. Its members appointed a committee which recommended major changes in the structure and physical plant of the Eastern Lunatic Asylum and the appointment of a qualified physician as superintendent. Much to Jarvis's discomfort the proposals to reorganize the hospital were defeated. "Economy was one objection," he observed, "and the unwillingness of the men of Lexington to have the system changed was another." In the face of mounting criticism both within and without the state, however, the legislature reversed its decision. By the spring of 1844 a physician had been appointed superintendent and renovation of the hospital's physical plant and changes in its operation were under way. Although Jarvis was no longer a resident of the state at the time, he was pleased with the outcome of his labors.[47]

If the state was responsible for the welfare of the insane, did it not have comparable responsibilities toward other dependent and distressed groups? Certainly this question had occurred to Jarvis by 1841. Although he had not yet developed a systematic approach to the resolution of social problems, he was not hostile to an expansion of public welfare. His vision of the political process, however, was such that he did not conceive of government as autonomous or merely representative of the views of its constituents. Public policy was to follow instead from the deliberations of objective, dispassionate, rational, and competent individuals whose conclusions were based upon careful analysis of empirical data. Blurring differences between values and data, Jarvis never envisioned that others holding alternative conceptual frameworks might reach fundamentally differing conclusions from the same set of data. The universe was too harmonious to permit such discrepancies; the proper role of the scientist involved the amassing of facts that would objectify moral preconceptions and demonstrate their validity.

When Samuel Gridley Howe, who was already famous for his work in educating the blind, toured the West and visited Louisville and Frankfort in an effort to persuade the legislature to appropriate $10,000 to establish a school for the blind, Jarvis joined a group of eminent citizens and threw his support behind the project. In establishing such an institution the state would fulfil its responsibility by helping those whose physical disability inhibited their full development as moral, intelligent, and productive citizens. Jarvis's enthusiastic letter to the *Boston Medical and Surgical Journal,* however, angered the editor of the *Western Journal of Medicine and Surgery* because it ignored strong indigenous support for the measure that antedated Howe's visit. In early 1842 the legislature passed a law establishing the Kentucky Institution for the Blind. Jarvis was immediately appointed a trustee, since he had been among those responsible for the passage of the law. His decision to return to Massachusetts ended his active role, but there was little doubt that his conception of social policy was beginning to emerge in its mature form.[48]

VII

During his years in Louisville, Jarvis was unable to adjust to new surroundings, despite his prominence in the community. He and his wife were received with gracious hospitality, but neither was comfortable in a state that retained a frontier character and lacked mature social relationships, cohesion, culture, and refinement. Above all, they found slavery hateful and, given its pervasive presence, unavoidable. Weariness with the prevailing monotony was relieved by an occasional visit to Concord. These trips, however, did not compensate for Jarvis's growing disillusionment with Louisville. Nor did an extended visit to his brothers Stephen and Nathan in New Orleans improve his outlook.[49]

Professional success might have compensated for dissatisfaction with Western society. But, much to his chagrin, Jarvis found that his medical practice was growing less and less successful. He was disturbed by the failure of people to pay their bills, especially those with sufficient resources. "I had no conception, that these people could so falsify their promise!" he observed. In five years his billings amounted to nearly $15,000 and his expenses to $4,700. Aside from repaying old medical school debts, he was unable to save; most of his income was represented in uncollected bills. Undoubtedly the severe business depression that began in 1837 was responsible for the inability of some to pay their debts. The transient nature of the city's population also made it impossible to turn over some delinquent accounts to collectors. Nor were his difficulties due to excessive charges. Compared with other physicians his fees were modest; he charged only one dollar per visit.[50]

Compounding the economic problem was the absolute decline in the number of individuals seeking his professional services. A diminishing income was one thing; a loss of patients was quite another, for it represented a bitter personal blow. Few physicians in Louisville had a comparable education; yet they succeeded where he failed. The doubts that plagued him first in Northfield and then in Concord now recurred even more intensely than before. "The more I observe, the more do I distrust myself as to my hopes of success in my profession," he wrote in anguished terms in his diary. "I dont know how it is, but it seems to me that success in treating cases did not gain for me other cases as it does for other men. It has seemed strange to me, that when people employ me, their friends or diseases are cured. They praise me, get others to employ me, & yet when they are sick again, they send for another physician." On one occasion he saved the lives of two individuals, but the family never again called upon his services.[51]

In early 1842 Jarvis learned from Howe that Dr. Samuel B. Woodward, the eminent superintendent of the Worcester State Lunatic Hospital in Massachusetts, was contemplating retirement. Still longing for a superintendency, he immediately wrote to Horace Mann, who had been responsible for the founding of the hospital in 1830 and subsequently had served as a trustee before becoming secretary of the State Board of Education. "I prefer," Jarvis observed, "that happy combination of the benevolent with the scientific, the exercise of the moral as well as the intellectual powers, in professional labour that is demanded in the treatment of lunacy, more than in ordinary business." Jarvis also looked forward to returning to New England, "where benevolence finds more sympathy than in the western country."[52]

Shortly thereafter Jarvis learned that Woodward had postponed his retirement, but that the position of assistant physician was vacant following the selection of Dr. George Chandler as head of the New Hampshire Asylum for the Insane. He immediately wrote to Woodward applying for the position. Unfortunately the position was filled even before the arrival of his letter. Woodward then advised Jarvis to apply for the superintendency of the New York State Lunatic Asylum at Utica, which was about to open; he also thought that the impending reorganization of the Kentucky Asylum offered still another opportunity. Jarvis followed up Woodward's suggestions, only to be greeted by the news that while his name would be submitted to the Utica trustees, the possibility of favorable action was remote because of the large number of candidates. Meanwhile he also contacted Dr. James Jackson, who replied in a pessimistic tone.[53]

As prospects for an institutional affiliation grew more remote, Jarvis's spirits sank. In June 1842 his inner crisis reached a climax. It was now twelve years since he had entered private practice; his three attempts to establish himself in different communities were abysmal failures. For an individual like Jarvis, an inability to succeed, especially in Louisville, was galling. He had served this Western community well, both as physician and philanthropist, but his contributions were unrecognized and unrewarded. In desperation he came to the conclusion that his only solution lay in securing a hospital superintendency. "I desire now of all things to go into an Insane Asylum as superintendent. I feel that that is my peculiar vocation & that I can be more happy & useful in it." A superintendency would bring economic security and place him in a position where his authority could not be undermined by fickle and insensitive patients and where he could finally apply his moral and scientific precepts to the treatment of disease. Still hoping that one of the mental hospitals in the Northeast would be seeking a new head, he impulsively decided to leave for Boston in July and spend about six weeks surveying various possibilities. If nothing came of the trip, he would return to Louisville. Despondent over events, he was uncertain about the future. On June 26 he made the final entry in his diary, which he never again continued. "Sometimes methinks I have a radical discontent in my spirit. I was not contented in Northfield from 1830 to 1832. I grew discontented in Concord during 1835–6. I am not contented here. What is my difficulty? Is it within or is it outward."[54] At this time Jarvis lacked an answer to his own question. But within a year his life would be radically altered. Out of his distress would come a new career that would finally bring him a measure of the success and recognition he had for so long craved. With success would also come psychic contentment; never again would doubt prove as threatening as it did in mid-1842.

A NOTE TO THE READER. After 1842 Jarvis never again kept a diary. Instead he began the practice of making copies of many (but not all) of his letters in a series of bound volumes. Unfortunately, the bulk of this correspondence, while invaluable, dealt with his public and professional career; it revealed little of Jarvis as a person. Even the letters that he wrote to his wife in 1860 on a journey abroad were impersonal; they were largely confined to descriptions of people and places (although his strong attachment to Almira was evident throughout). The remainder of this biography, therefore, focuses on his role and significance as a physician and statistician and includes little of his personal life, if only because the nature of the surviving sources mandates such an approach. Even his autobiography, which he wrote late in life, is largely a summary of his work and achievements.

3

A New Career

Jarvis's desire to return to Massachusetts in 1842 reflected both disillusionment with Louisville and romantic perceptions of his native state. His image of the harmonious and homogeneous nature of New England derived from his familiarity with small communities; before 1837, with the exception of medical school, he never experienced the vicissitudes of urban life. His subsequent sojourn in Louisville only reinforced a desire to resettle among cultured and refined people who would readily appreciate his interests and talents.

Reality, however, proved to be very different. By the 1840s Massachusetts, like other Eastern states, was undergoing profound changes that were altering its character. Population growth, urbanization, economic and technological change, and immigration of minority ethnic groups had all combined to transform traditional institutional arrangements and patterns of behavior. Few questioned the benefits of material progress, but many were concerned with the problems that accompanied rapid social growth. Increasingly Americans looked to new institutional arrangements to deal with such social problems as poverty, crime, dependency, and disease. Beneath essentially political questions lay more profound issues. In a rapidly changing world, what values ought to determine public policy and private behavior? Even if a moral consensus existed, how could it be embodied in public policy? And what if there were large groups that dissented from prevailing community opinion?

Whatever his expectations, Jarvis quickly found that the world of his youth was gone. Unlike some critics, he did not seek to restore a mythical past; his quarrel was not with material progress or affluence, neither of which he rejected.[1] His concern was rather with the ways people perceived problems and the institutional remedies they urged. Progress was not to be halted; it was to be guided in a particular direction. During the 1840s he slowly but surely defined his life-long work: the classification and collection of data that would illuminate the direction in which divine authority intended Americans to move. Combining the role of scientific investigator, moral teacher, and prophet, he would emerge as one of the early pioneers of what in the nineteenth century was known as social physics. In this venture he would join other Americans and Europeans who transformed simple statistical inquiry into a study of "the co-existence and sequence of social phenomena in correlation with the environing conditions of social life."[2]

I

On July 14, 1842, Jarvis and his wife left Louisville, presumably to survey opportunities in the East. On the way they visited with Thomas S. Kirkbride at the Pennsylvania Hospital for the Insane and Pliny Earle at the Bloomingdale Asylum in New York City, both of whom encouraged Jarvis to seek an institutional affiliation. Upon his arrival in Concord he learned that the superintendency of the Boston Lunatic Hospital (a municipal institution opened in 1839) was vacant. Jarvis immediately began to lobby in an effort to convince the members of the city council of his merits. Much to his chagrin, another physician received the appointment.[3]

After learning that Amariah Brigham had also resigned the superintendency of the Hartford Retreat, Jarvis made an effort to secure this vacancy. During a visit to Hartford he found what he interpreted as favorable sentiment for his candidacy. When he heard nothing further, he made anxious inquiries. Dr. George Sumner, a manager at the Retreat for many years, felt compelled to defend himself against rumors that he was unfavorably disposed; he insisted that his only concern was the protection of the welfare of patients. Shortly thereafter John S. Butler became the new superintendent. Jarvis reacted in a characteristic manner; he attributed his failure to the fact that his Unitarian affiliation was unacceptable in an area that was a stronghold of Trinitarianism.[4] In reality religious differences played no role in the decision, which was due instead to the poor impression that he made after returning to Massachusetts. "J. does not stand so well as when he returned from Kentucky," noted Luther V. Bell in commenting upon his candidacy. "The shewman's advice at a menagerie is not always malapropos 'Stand a little further back and you can see (and be seen!) just as well.'"[5]

Depressed by this turn of events, Jarvis busied himself with odds and ends while seeking to clarify his future plans. To return to Louisville was out of the question. After a chance conversation with several colleagues, Jarvis decided to settle in Dorchester, a rapidly growing community adjacent to Boston, and open a general practice while simultaneously treating insane persons in his home. In March 1843 he settled into rented quarters, and in June was joined by his wife.[6]

For the first time in his career Jarvis did not lack business. Initially he hoped to develop a general practice and treat a small number of mentally ill patients. Within a few years, however, his psychiatric practice became dominant. In 1845 he rented a larger house; during the 1850s he confined his practice to the care of eight or nine insane individuals (of whom three lived in his home and the other five or six in nearby residences). This type of practice proved personally gratifying and financially rewarding. Generally patients paid between ten and twelve dollars per week for Jarvis's medical services. Board was an additional six dollars. Families were also liable for the wages and board of a private attendant if one was required. Total charges ran as high as twenty-five or thirty dollars per week, a figure at least three to four times the cost of care in exclusive private hospitals. The high cost of care did not in any way discourage referrals, and Jarvis's reputation brought patients from families willing to spend large sums and perhaps avoid institutionalization. Indeed, he could afford to be selective and accept only cases able to benefit from his supervision.[7]

Jarvis's rather abrupt success in the light of three previous failures was probably due to the unique context of his practice rather than to any significant change in personality or modus operandi. In the first place, his practice was relatively novel and filled a void between the extreme of hospitalization and the absence of private outpatient psychiatric care. Second, few patients came from the adjacent neighborhood or had previous contacts with Jarvis; most were referred because of his general reputation as a leading psychiatrist. It was also unusual for Jarvis to care for the same patient more than once. Hence his earlier inability to retain the allegiance of patients was not a factor in his new setting. Finally, Jarvis's authoritative personality may very well have had a beneficial therapeutic effect upon patients requiring structure and guidance, thereby enhancing his professional reputation. Whatever the reasons, there is little doubt that the success which proved so elusive for more than a decade was now a reality.

Such a practice—which was virtually unique in the entire nation—had the virtue of providing Jarvis with time to pursue other activities and interests. Aside from statistical and psychiatric research, he was able to write, consult, and serve as an expert witness in legal proceedings. Admittedly, he continued to experience occasional difficulties in collecting bills; he also rendered services at reduced rates when need was demonstrated. Given the affluent nature of his patients, these exceptions did not seriously impair his total income. For the remainder of his career he never lacked financial security, and he and Almira left an estate valued at over $40,000—a substantial sum by the standards of that age.[8]

In his psychiatric practice Jarvis emphasized moral treatment. His disillusionment with heroic interventionist therapeutics made him receptive to the ideas of Bigelow and others who favored the healing role of nature. Even in general practice Jarvis relied on care, diet, and regimen. Similarly, he followed the basic principles of moral treatment in cases of insanity. Certain individuals, he insisted, could be treated more effectively in private homes than in hospitals, which, by virtue of their size, were more rigid and structured. Nevertheless, Jarvis did not hesitate to regulate the lives of his patients down to the smallest detail if he thought it advisable. He did not neglect diet, exercises, or acquaintances, and insisted on a right to limit visitation privileges. In the case of a depressed woman who never learned "regularity

& discipline of life'' Jarvis attempted to alter her behavioral pattern by emphasizing order and structure. In another case he wrote to a concerned parent that the daughter was making rapid progress "towards complete health & power of self control . . . . She is very contented, lively, & cheerful. She has a great variety of occupation & amusement. She rides, walks, visits, swings, plays, works & sees much company in the house. She has gained much power, but not enough to prevent her from falling back finally, if she should now be taken home & exposed to the scenes & associations, amidst which she became disordered, or if she should be subjected to rash experiment or unsuitable course of treatment.'' The basic goal of treatment, in other words, was to keep patients' minds "away from their delusions and vagaries, to calm their excitement, and raise them from their depression.''[9]

To be sure, Jarvis's practice was not without its problems. Like most hospital superintendents, he found it difficult to hire qualified attendants. His personal life was also complicated by the presence of patients. Almira, who played the major role in managing the household and supervising the daily routine, sometimes found that her health precluded continuation of such activities. Under such circumstances Jarvis, who understood her central role, immediately barred new cases until she recovered.[10]

II

Financial success gave Jarvis both the leisure and tranquility to pursue those activities that were most compatible with his interests. Beginning in the 1840s, therefore, he began to elaborate his views on the proper role of medicine. In 1843 he used the pages of the *Christian Examiner,* the famous journal of New England Unitarianism, to present his views. The immediate occasion was the publication of Horace Mann's sixth report as secretary of the Massachusetts State Board of Education, which urged that schools provide children with instruction about health. In this document Mann combined the perfectionist faith of nineteenth-century American Protestantism with the phrenological belief that environment, behavior, and physical development were indissolubly linked together. By this time

Massachusetts faced a variety of novel social and economic problems. Many of its citizens saw a causal relationship between the rising number of foreign-born, especially the Irish, and the increase in dependency, debauchery, and crime. How could this distressing state of affairs be changed? To individuals like Mann the answer lay in the establishment of a universal, free, and compulsory system of education capable of inculcating values among groups requiring socialization. The thrust toward public education during these decades, therefore, simultaneously reflected fear of the present and confidence in the future.

In reviewing Mann's report in a lengthy two-part article, Jarvis spelled out his own views. At the outset he explicitly rejected the popular belief that life was a "mystery"; that health was the gift of nature; and that diseases were God's punishment. Human beings were more than passive recipients of the means of life. Granting the absolute perfection of God's creation, Jarvis nevertheless insisted that men possessed the freedom to negate the divine gifts given them. Law, in other words, was the ethical standard by which humanity would be judged as well as a statement of the consequences that would follow a particular act. The concept of law as immutable and deterministic was anathema to Jarvis, since it was subversive of his religious faith and belief in free will. Evil was simply the consequence of unlawful or immoral behavior; the choices facing people were infinite. "God has put our lives, partially at least, into our own hands," he averred. "Whether we shall live to the fulness of our years, and give to each day its fulness of strength and pleasure, or whether we shall be miserable invalids, ever moving toward the grave and cut off in the morn, noon, or eve of life; these depend upon our obedience to those laws which God has stamped upon our frames."

Few people, however, lived their normal span of three score and ten years. Citing mortality figures from Boston and English registration reports, Jarvis demonstrated that average longevity was about thirty-five years, during which time the lives of many were further diminished by disease and disability. More than half the physical ills and deaths arose "from an ignorance of those laws of our being." The harmonious physiological processes of the human body would function efficiently if people followed proper diets, breathed pure air, exercised properly, and maintained a clean environment. The overwhelming majority of people, by way of contrast, lived amidst filth and pollution; they breathed air fouled by industrial fumes and tobacco; they substituted stimulants and narcotic beverages for water; they ate improper food and indulged themselves; they refused to bathe regularly and carried instead a "corrupting waste." Civilization, noted Jarvis, may have given rise to social refinements and mental pleasures, but it also promoted dissipation and diminished physical vitality.

The basic problem was not merely a general ignorance of the laws of life, but, among many, "a contemptuous disregard of them." Though these laws were indeed fixed and immutable, the "circumstances of life" were variable. "We believe," concluded Jarvis in words that spelled out the theme that would become the foundation of much of his subsequent work, "that if we would give the whole power of our intellect to learn the conditions of our existence, and our moral powers to fulfil them as correctly and as faithfully as we study the nature and watch the interests of our cattle, or our machinery, we should in a single generation be saved from many diseases, and very materially prolong life."[11] The attainment of health was not a utopian goal; its achievement required a judicious mixture of knowledge and wisdom. In political terms Jarvis's analysis presupposed that the major function of government was to educate its citizenry; he rejected an interventionist model that relied upon positive sanctions and coercion. Individual regeneration could only be achieved through voluntaristic appeals to the reason and sense of self-interest possessed by all human beings.

In expounding such views, Jarvis aligned himself with a relatively small but influential group of physicians and laymen who were convinced that the answer to social and medical problems (between which they did not distinguish) lay in preventive rather than curative techniques. In the absence of a demonstrable etiology or a specific germ theory of disease, they were led to interpret health as a consequence of a proper, virtuous, and orderly relationship between nature, society, and the individual. Disease followed the violation of the natural laws that governed human behavior and was indissolubly linked with filth, immorality, ignorance, and improper living conditions. Cities, especially those with large numbers of impoverished aliens, offered convincing evidence of this thesis. Such concepts were particularly suited to sanitary reform and general preventive measures, and they offered to Jarvis and other public health activists a means of reasserting the paramount importance of the medical profession in a changing world. The prevailing emphasis on the maintenance of health, therefore, reflected in part an inability to deal with disease per se—a fact that had impressed Jarvis since medical school. The thrust toward public health was further strengthened by the impact of French medicine and the application of Pierre Louis' numerical method, which tended to discredit traditional therapeutics.

For the remainder of his career Jarvis would elaborate and refine his belief in the prophylactic and didactic role of medicine. When informed in December 1848 that he had been chosen to deliver the annual address before the prestigious Massachusetts Medical Society the following spring, he selected this theme for his subject.[12] Medicine, he inferred, was too preoccupied with the cure of disease rather than the preservation of health. Indeed, physicians had neglected to define the attributes of perfect health, an understanding of which was indispensable if the body were to be returned from its "wanderings in the devious path of disease." Moreover, medicine had within its power the means to extend the normal life span of human beings. In raising these questions Jarvis was among those of his contemporaries who were holding out to their fellow countrymen the enticing prospect of greater longevity and freedom from disease.

In terms easily understood by physicians and laymen, Jarvis spelled out his philosophy and vision of medicine. The condition of human beings, he insisted, was related to the production of "vital force" (more commonly known as the "constitution" of man), which was "the aggregation of all the physical powers, the original organization, the united energies of the nutritive, respiratory, cutaneous, locomotive, and nervous actions, and the predominance of the vital over the chemical affinities." Only by the most faithful compliance with the laws of nature could men maximize the production of such force, for every deviation diminished and diluted its potency. The effect of errors, moreover, was cumulative. Thus sickness was prevalent "among the poor who must endure privations, among the weak and foolish who mismanage themselves, and among the wicked who abuse themselves."

By this time Jarvis was familiar with the work of leading English sanitary reformers, including Edwin Chadwick and T. Southwood Smith, as well as the growing body of social and medical statistics collected by governments concerned with health and mortality and by life insurance companies seeking a sound actuarial base for their policies. Appalled at the social costs of disease, sanitarians in many countries had begun to classify, collect, and analyze a vast body of aggregate data that would aid in formulating sound public policies intended to minimize the social and economic consequences of disease and poverty. Summing up their collected findings, Jarvis compared the incidence of sickness in various age groups and the average duration of life in different countries. Aware of differential mortality rates, he was even more impressed with the data that revealed high death rates in densely-populated regions as well as the close relationship of poverty with physical and mental morbidity and mortality. Even in the most favored regions—England and rural Massachusetts—relatively few individuals lived their normal life span; in the former 47 percent died before reaching the age of sixteen and in the latter 40 percent.

Why did mankind suffer such grievous and unnatural losses, asked Jarvis? To Chadwick the answer was clear; poverty and disease were products of industrialization and urbanization. Jarvis, on the other hand, was less interested in antecedent causes; he implied that all societies faced comparable social problems. His answer, therefore, was phrased in somewhat different terms. "There is a general ignorance of the laws of vitality," he told his colleagues. "Men do not understand the connection between their conduct and vital force; and they feel but little responsibility for the maintenance of health. They lay their plans and carry on their operations, without much regard to the conditions of their existence. Life and its interests are not always paramount considerations; but they are made subordinate to matters of inferior importance. They are sacrificed or made to yield to common conveniences and concerns." The widespread uses of tobacco and alcohol, improper diet and ventilation were but some of the elements that blocked the attainment of health. Worse still, the weaknesses of parents were transmitted to their offspring. While denying the feasibility of breeding human beings as cattle and horses were bred, Jarvis advised men and women to pay close attention to their prospective mates. In this respect the registration of births, deaths, and marriages played a vital role, for they provided accurate genealogical information.[13]

In "The Production of Vital Force" Jarvis offered a definitive statement of his mature medical philosophy.[14] In some ways his address was a reflection of his romantic attachment to Concord and his later experiences in Northfield and Louisville. Nor was his analysis particularly profound. He argued that violation of natural law produced disease, but at the same time he rejected determinism in favor of free will. He avoided altogether the philosophical problem of reconciling his faith in the freedom of the human will with his concept of an orderly and lawful universe. Perhaps his Unitarian upbringing and study of moral philosophy at Harvard solved the problem for him; perhaps his concrete mind never perceived the existence of such a problem. Whatever the reasons, he was disinterested in exploring abstract questions in depth; his mind was better suited for practical rather than theoretical problems. Having stated his general position, he looked forward to gathering the data that would fill in existing gaps in human knowledge. When Josiah Bartlett sought an appropriate subject for his address before the Massachusetts Medical Society, Jarvis advised him to speak on the uncertainty of medicine. The profession, Jarvis remarked, had to contend with inaccurate "vital & morbid & medical facts." This situation was related to a variety of factors: lack of exact knowledge of fundamental principles; failure to observe strictly; absence of a well-defined and universal nomenclature; failure to accumulate and coordinate the findings of all earlier and contemporary observers; and rash and hasty generalizations. The remedy was self-evident. Medicine had to discover its fundamental principles, articulate a universally valid nomenclature, and employ a "statistical use of facts so as to show the accumulation of all observations, and the results of every ones observations be added to the

sum of all others.'' Unconsciously or knowingly, Jarvis had out-
lined his life's work.[15]

In turning to statistical inquiry, Jarvis joined a small but influential group of individuals who not only were reorienting the
theoretical basis of medicine, but who were creating a new synthesis with important political and ideological consequences.[16]
During the 1830s and 1840s American scientists remained committed to the Baconian philosophy of science. Under this philosophy the ideal scientist began with a completely open and
unprejudiced mind, observed and collected a large number of
facts, and then deduced relevant laws. Conversely, speculation
and hypothesizing were pernicious activities that could only foster improper and erroneous views. In effect, Baconians adopted
a philosophy of rationalistic empiricism, which, if consistently
pursued, would lead to a full understanding of the universe.
The Baconian approach harmonized with the belief of Scottish
Common Sense philosophers that the senses and the mind could
perceive a real and objective external order. Hence accurate observation could not possibly give rise to erroneous facts. Error
could only arise by too hasty generalization or inadequate facts.[17]

The rationalistic empiricism of American science in turn created an extraordinary receptivity toward taxonomy. By the early
nineteenth century botanists, zoologists, and mineralogists were
in the vanguard of the movement to classify phenomena, and
physicians were already following in a similar direction. Indeed,
Linnaeus, who laid the foundation of modern taxonomy during
the eighteenth century, published a small volume in 1763 that
attempted to classify diseases. The underlying assumption of
taxonomical science was that genera and species had a natural
and independent existence apart from the subjective perceptions of the human observer. Just as plants could be classified, so
could diseases. The goal of nosological medicine, therefore, was
twofold: first, to give clear and precise definitions of diseases;
and second, to exhibit the relationships and inner nature of disease states by grouping together states with similar characteristics.[18] Once this was accomplished, it might then become
possible to identify the conditions that determined health and
disease. Unable to establish the etiology of diseases, physicians

began to develop a nosology of diseases based on external symptoms in the belief that they would be able to determine causation by employing a statistical methodology.

Nor was Baconian science or nosology inconsistent with a teleological interpretation of the universe; in this respect early nineteenth-century American medicine and science were not in conflict with Protestant Christianity. The orderly and rational nature of the universe was but a reflection of the work of a wise and beneficent Deity who had endowed biological creatures with a "vital force" that enabled them to achieve the purpose for which they had been created. Vague and ill-defined, the concept of a "vital force" was not necessarily inimical to the prevailing mechanistic interpretation of nature.[19] Defined in such a manner, Baconian science stimulated the thrust toward classification and data collection while leaving untouched other epistemological and ontological questions. By mid-century the Baconian approach was beset by increasingly troublesome dilemmas. But to individuals like Jarvis who had been reared and educated in a world that synthesized science, theology, and Common Sense philosophy, a life devoted to the development of an objective nosology and the collection of facts was entirely appropriate. For the remainder of his long and productive career he would concentrate on these activities, pursuing them even after the basic character of American science and medicine was sharply altered.

Admittedly, Jarvis's understanding of medicine was atypical; the overwhelming majority of practitioners were concerned more with patients than with theory, with cure than with prevention. Yet the structural context of mid-nineteenth-century medicine enhanced Jarvis's prominence and influence. At that time a profession was defined not by the possession of specialized knowledge, but by the character of its members. Oftentimes the debates that wracked medical societies reflected less a disagreement over the scientific qualifications of members than their personal attributes or character. For if medicine and science were inseparably linked with a moral and religious code, it was impossible to isolate knowledge within a separate compartment. Within this context the ideal physician combined knowledge with morality and social activism. These attributes were sometimes subsumed under the general heading "philanthropy," a term that not only defined a profession, but that also lay at the very center of antebellum society. Under these circumstances a profession could not function in an exclusionary manner. On the contrary, its members had an inescapable obligation to join with other individuals and groups who shared common values and whose character was above reproach in order to uplift society.

To a remarkable degree Jarvis embodied many of the intellectual, scientific, and religious currents of his age. Some of his contemporaries would turn to antislavery, others to temperance, world peace, education, women's rights, or a religiously based communitarianism, to cite only a few examples. In selecting medicine as a career Jarvis was no different from these individuals. Obviously medicine included, but was not limited to, the achievement of personal economic goals. But medicine was more than an occupation, for it unified knowledge with morality and religion. It was this very synthesis that gave to figures like Jarvis standing and influence. For if the origins of disease lay in either immoral or ignorant behavior, the remedy had to include more than simple medical intervention. To his fellow countrymen Jarvis brought a message of hope; implied in his career was the conviction that evil and ignorance could be extirpated by rational and moral human action. The generally friendly receptivity accorded Jarvis's emphasis on nosology and statistical inquiry (as well as his influence in helping to make quantified data the prerequisite for policy formulation) was a reflection of the widely held belief that these were but one side of a coin; on the other were imprinted moral and religious truths. And to remove either side was a logical and physical impossibility; one could no more conceive of a one-sided coin than one could interpret science and religion in antithetical terms.

III

By the time Jarvis settled in Dorchester, his fascination with nosology and data was clear. The precise direction that his future work would take, however, remained in doubt. Largely by accident he became embroiled in a controversy that would set the stage for his efforts to transform the nature of the federal censuses during the 1850s and 1860s.

Just prior to leaving Louisville in mid-1842, Jarvis's fascination with statistical materials led him to peruse the recently issued sixth census of 1840. Fifty-years old, the census had grown out of the provision in the federal constitution stipulating that political representation in Congress was partially dependent on population; hence some type of enumeration was required. While the idea of the census was by no means new, earlier censuses reflected a need for certain types of data by administrative and policy-making officials; the results of these inquiries often remained secrets of state. The first federal census in 1790 was restricted to a simple enumeration of population; the schedule listed only six questions. Between 1790 and 1830 there was a tendency to refine population statistics and on occasion add a manufacturing schedule. Gross administrative weaknesses, however, made the results of these censuses suspect. As American society confronted new social problems, the need by policy officials for accurate data multiplied. The census of 1840 reflected the growing interest in social statistics; its schedules included questions on population distribution, illiteracy rates, the number of educational institutions, and the total insane and mentally retarded ("idiotic") persons cared for by public funds. Aside from its use as a source of data, the census also appealed to nationalistic sentiment, since it seemed to offer proof that America was destined to become the predominant world power.[20]

Published in 1841, the sixth census was the first to provide some national statistics pertaining to the incidence of mental illness. There were, according to this compilation, over 17,000 insane and mentally retarded persons in the nation. Of these, about 14,500 were white and nearly 3,000 black. In the North the ratio of insanity among whites was 1:995; the comparable figure for the South was 1:945. Of the 2.7 million blacks in the South, 1,734 were insane or retarded, a ratio of 1:1558. In the free states, however, nearly 1,200 blacks out of a total population of 171,894 were insane or retarded, a ratio of 1:144. In other words, the census of 1840 purportedly demonstrated that the incidence of mental disease among free blacks exceeded that among slaves by nearly elevenfold and that among whites by six-fold.[21] The implications of these statistics, of course, were far-reaching. Indeed, a number of Southerners, including Secretary of State John C. Calhoun, immediately used this data to defend slavery and to justify territorial expansion.[22]

Jarvis first turned his attention to the census in a paper published in September 1842. Much of the article was devoted to a discussion of the inaccuracy of the statistics of insanity in the United States. Reports by local officials, he pointed out, generally revealed a far higher incidence of mentally ill persons within a given locality than did the federal census, and such local reports were usually the work of knowledgeable and informed men. The second half of the article discussed the great incidence of insanity among free blacks and the relatively low incidence among slaves. Jarvis was not particularly surprised at this finding, for it seemed to confirm the popular belief that the lower the state of civilization, the smaller the incidence of mental illness. It was natural for slaves—all of whom were insulated from excessive mental activity and the pressures of society—to show a low frequency of insanity as compared with their Northern counterparts occupying a "false social position." Nevertheless, he felt that further investigation of unknown variables was warranted. Additional research might prove that insanity was not necessarily the lot of cultivated men, especially if "advancing civilization may find means to anticipate all the evils attendant upon its progress, or ways to remove them if they cannot be prevented."[23]

After his initial article Jarvis continued to work through the census. Shortly thereafter he came to the frightening realization that there were gross errors in the official figures. The census volume, for example, listed 133 black insane paupers in the town of Worcester, Massachusetts, even though the total black population was only 151. Fearing other errors, he examined the statistics for each town in the Bay State and carefully compared the total black population with the number of black insane persons. The results were astounding; localities without any black residents were listed as having black insane individuals. Twenty-one towns with a total black population of twelve had, according to the census, no less than fifty-six black insane persons. Clearly, concluded Jarvis in a brief communication, the census was in error and should be corrected.[24]

Still dissatisfied, Jarvis was not content to let the matter rest. His sense of propriety was outraged, partly because his hope of using aggregate data in a scientific and objective manner had been dealt a staggering blow. Distressed too by the misuse of the census by proslavery advocates, Jarvis published a lengthy and detailed critique of the errors of the census in early 1844, showing that mistakes were not confined to black insane persons, but included whites as well. His essay closed with a broadside. The census, he proclaimed,

> has contributed nothing to the statistical nosology of the free blacks, and furnished us with no data whereon we may build any theory respecting the liability of humanity, in its present phases and in various outward circumstances, to loss of reason or of the senses. We confess, we are disappointed, we are mortified; nor are we alone in this feeling; our government had directed, that seventeen millions of people of various races and conditions, should be counted and their precise amount of derangement ascertained. Scientific men and philanthropists looked for the results of this investigation with confident hope; for henceforward the statistics of insanity, of deafness, and of blindness, were to be no more a mere matter of conjecture, but of positive and extensive demonstration. In due time the document came forth, under the sanction of Congress, and "corrected at the Department of State." Such a document as we have described, heavy with its errors and its misstatements, instead of being a messenger of truth to the world, to enlighten its knowledge and guide its opinions; it is, in respect to human ailment—a bearer of falsehood to confuse and mislead. So far from being an aid to the progress of medical science, as it was the intention of government in ordering these inquiries, it has thrown a stumbling-block in its way, which it will require years to remove.[25]

Ultimately Jarvis came to the conclusion that Congress had to repudiate the work of its own employees. Probably at the urgings of the sympathetic Henry I. Bowditch, Jarvis turned to the American Statistical Association for aid. Elected to membership in February 1844, Jarvis immediately introduced a resolution directing the organization to petition Congress to revise the published census. After the adoption of his proposal, he was appointed to the committee charged with implementing the resolution and then assigned the task of writing the actual text. At the same time he resumed his membership in the Massachusetts Medical Society and joined other members in an effort to discredit the statistics of insanity pertaining to the Bay State. His desire for action grew even stronger after he learned of Calhoun's use of the census data. "I little thought, when I wrote my pamphlet last fall," he told Dorothea L. Dix, "that so soon would the second officer of our nation make such use of the falsehoods of the census, and produce such an atrocious piece of sophistry as Mr. Calhoun has in regard to slavery & Texas."[26]

In February 1844, the dubious quality of the census became a matter of congressional concern when John Quincy Adams introduced a resolution directing the secretary of state to inform the House of Representatives if there were errors and what steps were being taken to rectify them. Calhoun responded by denying the existence of any inaccuracies. Meanwhile Jarvis and two other members of the American Statistical Association completed their memorial, which was sent to Congress in the late spring. Requesting remedial action, the petition noted that the census was deficient in a number of respects. The statistics on education were grossly inaccurate; the figures on the number of persons engaged in commerce were inconsistent and contradictory; and the data on the number of black insane persons were absurd. After making an intensive analysis, Jarvis and his colleagues concluded that the census did not deserve to have official sanction and they urged that it either be corrected or else repudiated.[27]

Despite prodding by Adams (one of the staunchest antislavery advocates in Congress), the House took no action on Jarvis's petition or a similar one sent by a group of antislavery Pennsylvanians led by Thomas Earle (brother of Pliny Earle, the eminent psychiatrist). The result was much the same in the Senate. Indeed, Calhoun seemed to add insult to injury when he sent a lengthy communication to the House in early 1845 defending the accuracy of the census and reaffirming his belief that slaves had a far lower incidence of insanity, blindness, deafness, and dumbness than free blacks. He also included a spirited defense of the integrity of the census written by William A. Weaver of the State Department, who attacked Jarvis and other critics for alleged misstatements of fact and other erroneous allegations. Admitting that the figures for Worcester represented an obvious blunder caused by the transposition of columns, Weaver insisted that there were errors on all sides which, taken in the aggregate, canceled each other.[28]

While seeking congressional action, Jarvis convinced *Hunt's Merchants' Magazine* to publish the entire text of the memorial in order to publicize the dispute. He was also gratified by the favorable notices given his efforts by some of the leading medical periodicals as well as expressions of support by colleagues. His efforts to secure remedial legislation, however, proved futile. Jarvis was of the opinion that the errors in the census were so useful to Southerners bent on annexing Texas and defending slavery that they could ill afford the luxury of permitting truth to prevail. Although his hopes for rectifying the injustice were all but obliterated by the larger controversy engendered by the Mexican War, he refused to let the matter rest. For over a decade he continued a virtual one-man crusade to secure repudiation of a document that made the American people "a laughing stock to all philosophers, for attempting to palm off upon the world such crudities in vital science." Had the census stated "that water ran up hill in the free states, and at various angles of elevation varying from the lowest in New Jersey to an elevation twenty times as great in Maine," he wrote to John Gorham Palfrey, "it would have contradicted the laws of natural philosophy no more than the statements, respecting the liability of the colored to mental disorder contradict the laws of pathology." When the *American Journal of Insanity* reprinted an article from a New York paper that used the census of 1840 as evidence of the inferiority of blacks, Jarvis wrote an angry rejoinder that repeated the substance of his earlier criticisms.[29]

Concerned less with injustices to blacks than with the accuracy of data, Jarvis slowly came to the realization that more than the exposure of error was required. In 1848 he persuaded the American Statistical Association to petition Congress to take the proper precautions to prevent any future repetition of the errors that plagued the census of 1840. Ultimately he concluded that such errors grew out of the very structure of the census itself. The original plan embraced too many items of inquiry. Moreover, incompetent persons whose only qualification was their political ties administered and directed the census. Only basic reforms would enable the census to fulfil its promise of providing the knowledge essential to the formulation of a proper and intelligent public policy.[30] In subsequent decades Jarvis would play a key role in creating the modern federal census.

IV

The amassing of objective data that would serve as the basis for the formulation of broad generalizations or laws was only one of Jarvis's ambitions as his new career pattern matured during the 1840s. Still another ambition was his desire to disseminate throughout American society a sure knowledge of the laws that governed human behavior. Aware of the profound forces that were undermining traditional institutions and patterns of behavior, he remained convinced that the social problems of a modern nation would be resolved through the application of reason and science, both of which would illuminate eternal moral truths. In one sense Jarvis spoke as an evangelical apostle of a new religion that made social science or political economy the partner of religious perfectionism. Ultimately the goal of all human institutions was the development of moral and regenerate individuals who, by virtue of strength of character, could not help contributing toward the creation of a just social order.

In the past American society had been forced to deal with the consequences of immorality, including insanity, indolence, crime, and delinquency. Policy at best was ameliorative and restorative in nature, for public authorities dealt with the activities of people whose careers were already flawed. To Jarvis, a policy directed toward the prevention of immorality was more rational and economical. In this respect he simply extended his faith in the prophylactic and didactic function of medicine to include nonmedical concerns. And the easiest way of preventing immorality was to ensure that social institutions produced moral and regenerate citizens who, by definition, would be incapable of improper behavior. There were, of course, many ways to maximize character. But the simplest and most obvious way was to make certain that individuals at birth would always be surrounded by proper influences. Certainly the family was paramount. But a significant auxiliary to the family was the school, which received children from a variety of environments, some good and others poor. Rightly structured, educational institutions possessed the capability of contributing to the building of character, particularly in cases where parents were morally deficient.

It was understandable, therefore, that Jarvis was attracted to Horace Mann, for the two had much in common. In preparing his sixth report as secretary of the Massachusetts State Board of Education, Mann consulted with Jarvis about the propriety of making physiology an integral part of the curriculum. Jarvis's favorable review of Mann's report further cemented the bonds between them. When Mann proposed that Jarvis prepare a textbook on physiology for use in the schools, the latter was more than willing. Here was a concrete opportunity to put his knowledge of medical science to practical use. The financial attractiveness of the project was also not lost on Jarvis, and by mid-1843 he decided to push ahead. Recognizing that the preparation of such a volume might take some years because of his unfamiliarity with the cognitive abilities of children, Jarvis declined to sign a contract with William B. Fowler and Nahum Capen of Boston and instead decided to complete the book before deciding upon a publisher.[31]

For the next three years Jarvis worked on the project. In 1845 he was invited to deliver a lecture in Hartford before the American Institute of Instruction (one of the early organizations devoted to spreading the gospel of education), and he used this forum to offer some of his ideas in preliminary form. The function of a common school education, Jarvis informed his listeners, was to teach children to read and write, and to study such subjects as geography, arithmetic, grammar, history, and science. But the responsibilities of schools toward their students went beyond these tasks. Individuals were "appointed to live" by their Creator, who granted to humanity life and the laws that governed life. Repeating the theme that was now an integral part of his outlook, Jarvis insisted that "health, vigor, and protracted life" followed "the faithful obedience to these laws," while "the melancholy consequences of pain and weakness, of sickness and premature death" followed from neglect and disregard of them. The moral was obvious: schools had an inescapable obligation to provide students with instruction in physiology. Such instruction was not to be confined to discussions of the structure and functions of vital organs and processes, but would include lessons on diet, clothing, exercise, and cleanliness. Nor were mental processes to be disregarded. For if the brains of young children were overtaxed, failure and weakness would inevitably follow and ultimately end in insanity. Citing a range of statistics that seemed to prove his case, he noted that the "wealthy and intelligent" lost between two-sevenths and one-half of their normal life span, while the comparable figure among the poor ranged between one-half and four-fifths. While Jarvis generalized from his own values, he was unwilling to exempt any group from his searching critique. Well-to-do as well as poorer groups stood to benefit from a strict observance of the laws of physiology, although the latter would benefit the most.[32]

In the spring of 1847 Jarvis was nearing completion of his book on physiology. Concerned with securing the widest possible distribution, he approached the reputable Philadelphia firm of Thomas, Cowperthwait & Company. Within weeks a contract was signed. Under its terms Jarvis paid for setting the plates, and the publishers assumed responsibility for printing and distribution costs. The four-hundred-page volume had a list price of eighty-eight cents, and Jarvis agreed to a royalty of nine cents per copy. Shortly thereafter Jarvis began to solicit endorsements, hoping that they would stimulate sales.[33]

Practical Physiology for the Use of Schools and Families was precisely what its title implied—a manual designed to provide intelligent readers with an understanding of complex human physiological processes. Such knowledge, if put to proper use, would enable individuals to lead full and happy lives free from disease, debility, and tragedy. Balance, emphasized Jarvis, was the key to health. "As in the perfect body all the organs are equally attended to, and all the muscles exercised, so in the perfect mind all the mental and moral faculties are developed, exercised, and strengthened, in due proportion." Mental and physical fitness and discipline gave human beings "command of their resources, and great power in every emergency." Individuals with fully developed adaptive mechanisms were capable of meeting all challenges no matter how severe. Implicitly Jarvis defined health as the ability to respond in a creative and efficient manner to the physical and social environment; those persons lacking adaptive traits would show higher morbidity and mortality rates. When expenditure exceeded income, the result was deterioration. Improper diet, lack of exercise, overexertion, and the use of alcohol and tobacco, for example, all destroyed the delicate balance between expenditure and income. "Each one of these errors," Jarvis warned, "diminishes the capital of life in proportion to its extent. One takes a little, and another a little, and yet the loss is unnoticed until the whole, added together, weakens the constitution, impairs the health, and wastes the strength so much, that some other cause creates a perceptible disorder or pain, and this we call *disease*."[34]

Although written for a didactic purpose and colored by his own moral and religious assumptions, Jarvis's *Practical Physiology* was for the most part a straightforward description of physiological processes as then understood. The book was divided into seven parts. The first covered digestion and food; the second the circulatory system and its role in nutrition; the third the respiratory system; the fourth the heat mechanisms of the body; the fifth the skin; the sixth the bone and muscular structure and the basic requirements for their effective functioning; and the final section discussed the brain and nervous system. Throughout Jarvis demonstrated a familiarity with recent medical literature; his discussion of the nervous system, to cite one illustration, was based upon William Beaumont's observations that gastric digestion was a predominantly chemical process. Moreover, Jarvis was not at all averse to identifying issues for which there were as yet no clear answers. Although he believed that a vegetarian diet was inferior to one that included meat, he conceded that there was no evidence that the former was injurious.[35]

Especially significant about *Practical Physiology* was its omission of any mention of the medical profession. Implicitly, Jarvis may have been expressing part of his disillusionment with traditional medical practice; he remained unconvinced that therapeutic intervention (with the possible exception of surgery) could appreciably alter the course of a disease. This being the case, logic dictated a preventive approach.[36]

Shortly after the publication of Jarvis's book, the prestigious *American Journal of the Medical Sciences* printed a favorable review.[37] Although pleased, Jarvis recognized that the length of the book and the level of writing rendered it unsuitable for younger children. By the spring of 1848 he had completed a much briefer and simplified version for use in the nation's common schools. Less than one-third the length of the original, the new book was published by the same firm. Jarvis had a twofold purpose in producing the brief version. Above all, he felt the necessity for providing children with adequate instruction in physiology in order to help them avoid any temptation that might adversely affect their development. But Jarvis was also mindful of the potential market for such texts. In his own mind both considerations merged, and he launched a determined campaign to promote his book.[38]

The first target Jarvis chose was Boston. Friendly with Horace Mann, Samuel Gridley Howe, and George B. Emerson—the three most influential figures on the local educational scene—he was hopeful of persuading the school committee to adopt his text. The moment appeared opportune, for in 1847 the Visiting Committee (of which Emerson was a member) strongly supported the introduction of "moral instruction," a subject that presupposed the study of physiology. By 1848 only a few schools had complied, but the prospects for full implementation in the fall semester seemed bright. A delay in printing the *Primary Physiology* led the school committee to adopt instead a similar book by Dr. Calvin Cutter, an action that infuriated Jarvis. His hostility notwithstanding, there were in reality few significant differences between the two books. Like Jarvis, Cutter based his book upon the principle of prevention and deemphasized the role of the physician in treatment, preferring instead to rely on "the natural powers of the system."[39]

Jarvis immediately set to work to persuade the school committee to reverse its decision. Not content to attack Cutter as a business rival, he denounced both the quality of the competing book and the tactics employed by its author.[40] Jarvis's goal of monopolizing the Boston market for his text, however, was never realized. Relatively few schools offered instruction in physiology; those that did generally had unhappy experiences. At the end of 1849 John Codman, chairman of the school examining committee, was blunt in his negative evaluation and suggested that the teaching of physiology be abolished. Jarvis immediately sent a letter of protest to Codman. In early 1850 the school committee dropped its specific endorsement of Cutter and voted a general recommendation of any book. Jarvis hoped that this action might provide an opening wedge and offered to forego royalty payments in order to reduce his book's price if this would facilitate its adoption. Shortly thereafter the legislature passed a law stipulating that schools should teach physiology and hygiene when school committees "shall deem it expedient." But continued experience with the subject was disheartening, leading the committee to urge its abolition.[41]

Nor was Jarvis's failure to capture the Boston market matched by large sales elsewhere. "I must confess," he told his publisher in 1854, "that hitherto the sale of these books has fallen short of my expectations." Between 1847 and 1855, 15,000 copies of the *Practical Physiology* were printed, and between 1848 and 1853, 10,000 copies of the *Primary Physiology,* most of which were sold. Jarvis, on the other hand, had hoped for an annual sale of between five thousand and seventy-five hundred of each. Certain that his books were superior, he could not understand the lack of public enthusiasm and constantly hounded his publisher in the hope of stimulating larger sales. His disappointment was further compounded by the fact that his royalties did not exceed the costs he incurred in setting the book in type.[42]

In 1856 the publishing firm of Thomas, Cowperthwait & Company failed, and for nearly six years Jarvis was unable to get a statement of sales or to recover the plates. After several years of intensive searching he managed to regain possession of the plates, but never received a precise accounting of sales. In 1865 the New York firm of A.S. Barnes brought out a slightly revised edition using the original plates. The changes in the new edition were minor. Only inconsequential discoveries had been made since 1847, Jarvis informed his publisher, and most of these were of a technical nature and of little interest to the public. Having grown to maturity in a different milieu, he did not appreciate the degree to which pathology was being transformed by figures like Theodor Schwann and Rudolf Virchow. Jarvis's world was of an entirely different character, a world dominated by religious and moral concerns. Disease was never an impersonal or strictly objective phenomenon; it usually followed in the wake of willful or unknowing disobedience to divine laws. Nor could physiological processes be divorced from the moral order. The interest in and importance of sanitary science, Jarvis noted, made his books even more relevant in the mid-1860s than they were at the time of their original publication. In the succeeding decade both books had steady though unspectacular sales.[43]

Although his experiences as an author were less than happy, Jarvis never abandoned his faith in the didactic function of medicine. If anything, his failure to make instruction in physiology and hygiene an integral part of the curriculum served as a catalyst, for the seeming increase in disease and mortality in the antebellum and postbellum periods simply demonstrated the magnitude of the task facing medical and sanitary science. Failure on one front was no reason for despair. Curiously enough, he remained somewhat oblivious of his school audience, which by the 1850s was composed of substantial numbers of children from poor and immigrant families. He believed in the importance of adequate diet, proper clothing, and decent housing, but never asked whether families had sufficient means for such necessities. If problems did exist, they were largely due to individual rather than structural defects; for all of his involvement with aggregate data, Jarvis defined the issue in terms of individual volition. Although he conceded on occasion that society, "in great degree, [is] responsible for the deficiency & error of members," his solution was revealing. The duty of society, he wrote, was "to relieve" the suffering and "to establish means of prevention." Education, broadly defined, played a vital role: it would develop man's faculties in due proportion; it would "repress & discipline the exuberant [and] the sensual"; it would promote a disciplined intellect and "energize & give supremacy

to the moral''; it would provide a "philosophy of life" and ensure the dominance of the conscience.[44] A moral people whose
behavior was determined by reason rather than passion could
not help but bring about the environmental transformation that
would reduce morbidity and mortality.

4

Vital Statistics and the Social Order

As Jarvis's medical philosophy and social ideology matured after his return to Massachusetts, he was forced to confront two basic issues. First, were existing nosological and classification systems adequate? Second, what was the quality of the collected data? If either or both were deficient, erroneous generalizations might follow. In turn, the general welfare might be impaired by the adoption of improper public policies by state officials who relied on the findings of physicians and scientists. Beginning with his analysis of the deficiencies of the census in 1840, Jarvis slowly intensified his efforts on behalf of proper classification and collection of accurate statistics, upon which all enlightened and benevolent public policies rested.

To figures like Jarvis the need for reliable data seemed even greater in the 1840s than at any time in the past. By then a rapidly burgeoning urban population and economic and technological changes created what seemed to be serious threats to health. In cities poorly ventilated and ill-conceived tenements exposed inhabitants to a host of dangers. Urban crowding, moreover, led to sanitary problems that grew out of inadequate means of sewage disposal, burial of the dead, and reliance on polluted water supplies. The rapid influx of immigrants like the Irish—who supposedly lacked the desirable attributes possessed by the native population—merely compounded the threat to the maintenance of a moral and therefore healthy society. The alarming increase in crime and pauperism that followed the migration of the Irish as well as their high morbidity and mortality rates added to the dangers threatening the very fabric of American society.

Committed to a partially mechanistic view of the relationship between behavior and disease, Jarvis concluded that priority had to be given to the collection of a vast body of reliable and significant observations, from which appropriate conclusions could be deduced. The collection of such data, however, was clearly beyond the capabilities of any single individual or group. Only public agencies whose power was derived from specific statutory authority were capable of undertaking such a task in a systematic and comprehensive manner. During the 1840s, therefore, Jarvis devoted considerable time and energy in efforts to convince state governments that it was in their best interest to create an agency to oversee the systematic collection of data. As a result of his endeavors, Jarvis became one of the most important spokesmen for improved registration and sanitary measures within Massachusetts and an influential figure on the national scene.

I

Jarvis knew that his influence as an individual was limited. If his dream of a healthy and moral social order was ever to become a reality, he would first have to find an institutional base in order to make his views known and thereby influence public policy. Political organizations rarely appealed to him; he was repelled by their opportunistic and expedient nature. Medical organizations, by way of contrast, had few liabilities and many advantages. This was particularly true of the Massachusetts Medical Society, one of the oldest and most distinguished bodies of its kind in the nation. Such was its authority that it was able to inhibit the rapid proliferation of medical schools in the Bay State, a development that elsewhere created serious friction between state medical societies seeking licensing authority and medical school proprietors seeking unrestricted acceptance of the M.D. degree as the only requirement for practice.

In 1833 Jarvis was elected a fellow of the society, but during the succeeding decade his involvement was nominal. Upon his return to Massachusetts in 1842 he took a more active role in its affairs. He was on various occasions elected as a counsellor and played a prominent part in the governance of the organization.

As a result of this affiliation, he attended some of the early meetings of the American Medical Association, where he spelled out his case for the adoption of a uniform nosology and the need for accurate observations. Most significant, Jarvis convinced the Massachusetts Medical Society to support several of his own projects within the Bay State.[1]

While membership in the society proved valuable and rewarding, Jarvis found that it did not meet all of his requirements, if only because the bulk of its membership was concerned with practice rather than research or theory. Fortunately, Jarvis soon found an ideal substitute in the American Statistical Association. Founded in 1839 by a small group of prominent Bostonians, the association served as a convenient meeting place for those interested in statistical knowledge. In the early days Lemuel Shattuck was its most important member, and he used the association as a means of building support for the adoption of an accurate and effective system of registration in Massachusetts. Nevertheless, the organization was little more than a small club; it often had difficulty in convening a quorum for its regular meetings. After becoming a member in early 1844, Jarvis began to use the association as an institutional source of support for a variety of projects beginning with his abortive effort to induce the federal government to renounce or correct the census of 1840. In 1847 he was elected vice-president, and in 1852 was elevated to the presidency, a position he retained for thirty-two years. For most of his presidency the association was largely his personal instrument to promote the cause of vital statistics. Because of its relatively small size, Jarvis was able to direct its activities as he saw fit. Although he professed disappointment with the association in his autobiography, the fact of the matter was that he did little to change its structure or alter its activities; to do either might have weakened his hold over its affairs.[2]

II

While creating an organizational base and working to correct the federal census, Jarvis turned his attention to the role of vital statistics in furthering public health. Jarvis, of course, was not alone in urging that social research should become the foundation of public policy. By the mid-1840s the work of English sanitarians, especially Edwin Chadwick, was well known in the United States. Chadwick first rose to fame during the inquiry of the Royal Commission appointed to study the operations of the Poor Laws between 1832 and 1834. Serving as a resource person to the commissioners, Chadwick virtually forced them to abandon any a priori study of the English welfare system. Legislation had to be founded upon ample deduction; any proper inquiry rested on a bedrock of hard facts. Rejecting orthodox laissez-faire principles, he argued that positive governmental action could alleviate, if not eliminate, many of the prevailing social problems that accompanied industrialization and urbanization. Pauperism, as he put it, was not a pathological entity undermining the structure of society, but simply a disorder of its functions that could be corrected by informed action. Eschewing speculative theories and utopian reforms, he insisted upon the paramount importance of comprehensive social investigations. Before the age of thirty he already had adopted the cardinal principle of the mid-nineteenth-century public health movement; namely, that the length and healthiness of life were determined by the circumstances in which people lived. His classic *Report on the Sanitary Condition of the Labouring Population of Great Britain* in 1842 was largely an elaboration of this principle. Like many of his contemporaries, he emphasized the superiority of preventive rather than remedial policies, and insisted that the community as a whole could only benefit from the destruction of festering slums, the diminution of crime, the increase of life expectancy, and greater productivity. Mortality and sickness, he proclaimed, were preventable by positive action—an idea that became a rallying point of sanitarians everywhere.[3]

The impact of Chadwick's work was felt both in Europe and the United States. Indeed, mid-nineteenth-century sanitarians were unconcerned with strictly national political boundaries, for they shared common assumptions about the relationship between environment and disease. Consequently, they attempted to forge an international scientific community that would facilitate the exchanges of experiences and knowledge that illuminated the links between industrialization and urbanization on the one hand and morbidity and mortality on the other. They were also cognizant of the international nature of epidemic diseases (especially cholera) and the futility of pursuing isolationist policies that ignored events elsewhere in the world.

In 1843 Chadwick published a supplementary report to the study of the English laboring classes that dealt with interment in towns. Just as urban residents lacked adequate housing accommodations, so Chadwick found that graveyard space was insufficient, particularly in urban areas. Emanations from human remains threatened "to produce fatal disease, and to depress the general health of whosoever is exposed to them." Chadwick's recommendations were simple, but radical for his day. He proposed that cemeteries be prohibited in residential areas; that the government provide public burial grounds and low-cost funerals; that health officers supervise burials; that no burial take place without verification of the fact and cause of death; and that in all cases of death "from removable causes of disease," health officers be given the authority to order the removal of these causes.[4]

In his published summary of Chadwick's report of interment, Jarvis accepted the cardinal tenet of public health activists; namely, that the duration and condition of life reflected environmental circumstances. In urban areas in particular the threat of "over-accumulation of the dead among the living" was menacing. Congestion in cities, warned Jarvis, was reaching the danger point. "In as far as we permit the putrefactions of the body to take place in our midst, to however small extent, we are violating those plain laws of life which require the air we breathe and the water we drink to be free, not only from all noxious intermixtures, but from all foreign ingredients whatever." Although failing to endorse any specific remedies, Jarvis closed his review with Chadwick's summary of burial procedures in Frankfort, Germany.[5]

An exponent of the utility of social research, Jarvis was not prepared to concede that Chadwick's vision of an active and interventionist government was required for the creation of a better society. Several months after his favorable piece on Chadwick, he published an equally long review of the new edition of Robley Dunglison's *Human Health*.[6] Expressing agreement with

Dunglison's general views about the influence of climate and living patterns on human health, Jarvis devoted much of his article to a summary of the data. Nevertheless, he was not inclined to endorse Dunglison's favorable impressions of the role of federal and state governments in promoting happiness and prosperity. In his critique he spelled out some of his own conceptions of the proper function of government, which differed from those of Chadwick or even John H. Griscom, whose *Sanitary Condition of the Labouring Population of New York* in 1845 paralleled the analysis and recommendations of his English counterpart. American governments, insisted Jarvis, had done little to prevent social problems; they "legislated for property, but not for life." Congress, for example, passed laws to increase productivity and supported studies to promote economic well-being, but avoided any study of the human costs that were involved.

In arguing in such terms Jarvis by no means supported positive legislation to promote the general welfare. What he proposed instead was a vast expansion of government data-gathering activities. His social and political assumptions remained individualistic, for he believed that scientific knowledge would create regenerate individuals who, by definition, would behave in a moral and lawful manner. Massachusetts, he wrote, was the only state that provided for the registration of births and deaths and the causes of mortality, and even its system was imperfect. Nor was the record of the federal government any better, as the census of 1840 demonstrated. A careful analysis of vital statistics, he insisted, demonstrated "that there is, at least, a field of inquiry almost untouched in America, but which we commend to the paternal care of our government to investigate and ascertain the extent of the evils."

In closing his review, Jarvis took Dunglison to task for citing a long list of literary and scientific figures who lived to old age. Such antiquarianism was dangerous and proved nothing. What Dunglison should have done was to compare the total number of individuals engaged in such callings with the experiences of other occupational groups. Only then would it have been possible to study the relationship between occupation and longevity.[7] Such criticisms were as revealing of Jarvis's concept of statistical research as they were of Dunglison's disregard of methodology.

Jarvis, as he would demonstrate consistently throughout his entire career, tended to assume that a statistical relationship implied causality. The phenomena that he chose to compare often reflected the values and moral outlook of his social class.[8]

During the 1840s Jarvis's belief in the paramount importance of vital statistics grew even more powerful. Slowly but surely he broadened his concerns to include a multiplicity of factors that influenced health and longevity, including climate, occupation, class, ethnicity, race, sanitary and environmental conditions, and personal behavioral traits. All had to be systematically observed and aggregated if they were to reveal in precise terms the natural laws governing mankind. Besides writing reviews of Chadwick and Dunglison, he received Harvard's prestigious Boylston Prize for his dissertation on the relationship between climate and longevity (although he failed in an effort to find a publisher for this work). Recognition came too from foreigners, one of whom presented to the Statistical Society of London some of Jarvis's statistical findings on the age distribution of the American population in different latitudes and mortality rates in selected areas.[9]

One individual, no matter how prolific, could not carry the burden of statistical research alone, and Jarvis was no exception. By 1844 he had helped to convince the Massachusetts Medical Society and the American Statistical Association to lobby for more effective governmental data-gathering procedures. Jarvis hoped to improve the quality of the data collected in Massachusetts, the most advanced state in the country, and also to persuade other states to follow suit. As early as 1639 the Massachusetts General Court had mandated that a record be kept of every birth, marriage, and death in the colony. Honored more in the breach than in the observance, the law nevertheless set a precedent, and interest in statistics was maintained during the seventeenth and eighteenth centuries. It must be noted that pre-nineteenth-century concern with registration did not reflect a desire to use such data for policy purposes or for health and population-related research. Vital events were registered instead in order to preserve the community's history and for use in legal matters related to probate and responsibility for paupers. By the beginning of the nineteenth century the concept of registration was undergoing fundamental changes as the realization grew that data and policy could have a symbiotic relationship. This change was strengthened by developments in England and on the continent, where statistical societies proliferated and the cause of social research was given impetus by figures like Quetelet and others. To nations facing the necessity of adjusting to novel social and economic problems, the need for systematic and accurate data was magnified. To an astonishing degree, the paramount position of the nation-state was based, at least in part, upon its capacity to gather data in a systematic and aggregate form. The cosmopolitan character of Massachusetts ensured that some of its citizens were informed about foreign developments.[10]

The most prominent figure in pushing for improved registration and census procedures in Massachusetts was Lemuel Shattuck, a former resident of Concord whose classic history of that town emphasized vital statistics.[11] An extraordinarily pietistic individual, Shattuck wanted to illuminate the grand design of nature by collecting and analyzing records and then deducing operative natural laws. After moving to Boston in 1837, he prepared an analysis of the vital statistics of the city from 1810 to 1841 that purportedly demonstrated that the sharp decline in health and rising mortality rates were the result of the adverse influence of urbanization and of changes in the simple style of life that in the past had fostered the maintenance of health. Subsequently Shattuck compiled a city census of Boston in which he warned of the dangers posed by the large number of immigrants living amidst squalid and crowded surroundings. Several years earlier he convinced the newly established American Statistical Association to press the Massachusetts General Court to enact a more effectual statute for the annual registration of births, marriages, and deaths. Shattuck's plan was based on the assumption that systematic records would lead to a better understanding of the relationship between the physical and moral order, thereby illuminating issues of public policy. Following the passage of the Registration Act of 1842, he continued the fight for more effective procedures in order to enhance the quality of the data that was being accumulated.[12]

After he returned to Massachusetts in 1842, Jarvis's interest in registration intensified. ''We need much to be done there—,'' he wrote to Horace Mann in an effort to enlist his support, "to show the people, by record & by document, how much, in what manner & in what places, they come short of their earthly destiny." Isaac Ray, already one of the nation's most prominent psychiatrists, urged Jarvis to pursue his studies of vital statistics, a subject too long neglected. Needing little encouragement, Jarvis became active in the Massachusetts Medical Society, which, like the American Statistical Association and the American Academy of Arts and Sciences, had been pressing the legislature to adopt more effective procedures.[13]

At its annual meeting in 1843 the society adopted a broad resolution dealing with the registration of diseases and their coexisting circumstances. Jarvis was appointed to a committee with John D. Fisher and Oliver Wendell Holmes. Taking cognizance of differential longevity and disease rates in their state, the three physicians urged the society to enlist the aid of members to keep records of data within their reach. In a longer report Fisher agreed with Jarvis that the medical profession was too preoccupied with the treatment of disease and had paid insufficient attention to prevention.[14]

After the members accepted their report, Jarvis, Holmes, and Fisher were appointed to a committee charged with the task of devising a plan to implement these proposals. Their report in turn urged member physicians to provide accurate descriptions of the topography and climate of their areas and to keep detailed statistical records for one year. They also recommended the adoption of the nosology developed by Dr. William Farr in England and used by that nation's Registrar-General.[15] Comprehensive in scope, the committee's report bore Jarvis's imprint, for it included a model questionnaire whose results could be easily aggregated. Indeed, it is likely that the draft was prepared by Jarvis.

Little came of this venture; few physicians had either the time or the inclination to keep detailed records, especially when the element of compulsion was absent. Disappointed by the paucity of results, Jarvis was unwilling to abandon the fight for more accurate data. By this time he had emerged as a leading member of a small but influential group that made sanitary reform the overriding objective of American medicine. Disillusioned with traditional therapies, its members insisted that the basic goal of medicine was the adoption of social measures that would promote community health by preventing disease. In 1846 Griscom introduced two resolutions at the first meeting of the National Medical Convention (which would shortly become the American Medical Association) that embodied the basic approach of sanitary activists. The first urged states to adopt more effective registration systems; the second called upon the profession to agree on a nomenclature of diseases in order to enhance the utility of registration categories. The convention approved both proposals and agreed to establish two committees, the first to prepare a report on registration and the second to draft a common nomenclature. Although not present, Jarvis was appointed to the second committee along with Griscom (chairman), Shattuck, T.R. Beck, Charles A. Lee, and Gouverneur Emerson.[16]

The following year Griscom's committee submitted a report entirely consistent with the views expressed earlier by Jarvis in the Massachusetts Medical Society. "A uniform and systematic plan of *registration* and *classification*," its members told the assembled delegates, "is essential to ensure this accuracy." The absence of a clearly stipulated nomenclature was an insuperable barrier; often the same disease went under a variety of names; and accurate comparisons of the prevalences of disease or the health of the population in different places and periods were impossible. The committee proposed that such subjective terms as "sudden," "acute," and "chronic" be dropped; that more precise categories be adopted; and that causes of death be certified by competent physicians. Its members then endorsed the classification system prepared by Farr.[17]

Farr's system summed up a good part of the medical and sanitarian thought of the mid-nineteenth-century. First, he made the classification of disease the prerequisite of further medical progress. Second, he took for granted the belief that disease was as much of a social as a medical problem. Finally, he insisted that changes in the urban environment could alleviate or diminish disease. Together these three assumptions formed a coherent and influential system. A proper nosology made possible the collection and analysis of data on disease, which in turn could be related to environmental factors. The results would enable government to take actions that were required to reduce or to eliminate those maladies that were so destructive of human life.

Between 1839 and 1880 Farr served as superintendent of the statistical department of the General Register Office, where he became the primary architect of the British system of vital statistics and a recognized world authority. Like most sanitarians, Farr was primarily interested in what was then designated as "zymotic" diseases, or epidemic, endemic, and contagious diseases, which taken as a group accounted for a significant proportion of total deaths. Farr's own explanation of the causes of disease seemed convincing, for it was buttressed by an impressive array of statistics. He argued that the introduction of specific zymotic materials (nonliving organic substances) into the bloodstream led to disease, since these materials were able to reproduce themselves. A simple contagion theory could not by itself explain the rapid spread of disease, and Farr insisted that most zymotic material was transmitted through the atmosphere. While temperature, humidity, and other climatic conditions played a role, the most significant elements were locally produced organic pollutants called miasmata, which aided in the formation of zymotic material. For all intents and purposes, then, squalor and dirt could cause disease, and Farr urged the adoption of measures to inhibit the formation of miasmatic material. This theory helped to overcome gaps in explanations that emphasized contagion and could account for the failure of quarantine to halt cholera epidemics. Moreover, it provided an adequate explanation for high urban mortality rates. Farr's theory of disease and his nosology found a champion in Jarvis, who intensified his efforts to improve registration systems and to convince the medical profession to adopt the Englishman's nosology.[18]

III

While working with Griscom's committee, Jarvis gave several papers at the meetings of the American Statistical Association that reflected his concern with vital statistics. He could not help being aware of the inadequacies of Bay State registration statistics, since Shattuck had so fully documented them in his analyses of the reports of 1843 and 1845.[19] Toward the end of 1847 Jarvis read a paper on vital statistics to the members of the American Statistical Association. Immediately thereafter the organization appointed a committee composed of Shattuck, Jarvis, and three other members to memorialize the Massachusetts legislature and request the appointment of commissioners to conduct a sanitary survey of the state. By January Jarvis had completed a draft based upon his paper, which was approved by the association and forwarded to the general court. As the result of some persistent lobbying, a large number of copies were printed and given wide circulation.[20]

The memorial reflected Jarvis's preoccupation with the circumstances that influenced human life. European governments, he pointed out, frequently conducted sanitary surveys in order to improve health and diminish disease. Could not Massachusetts act in a similar manner? The fact that the duration of life varied so significantly within the state provided conclusive evidence that environment and disease were intimately related. How else could variations in mortality rates between counties be explained, to say nothing about differences between socioeconomic groups within the same county? The government, he continued, already promoted economic development, often ignoring its adverse consequences for health. Did it not have an equal obligation to prevent further diminution of health? The state constructed dams in order to provide an abundant power supply for its burgeoning factories, which in turn created new jobs. Yet little attention was paid to the effect on human life by the transformation of the environment or the creation of new occupations.

Economic development, moreover, fostered urbanization, and there was a growing body of data to show that density of population was directly proportional to diminished vitality and higher mortality rates. The available evidence also disputed the popular conviction that Americans enjoyed a longer life span than other peoples and that this span was increasing. As a matter of fact, the average longevity in Massachusetts was less than in Sweden, France, and some counties in England, and it was, contrary to popular belief, growing shorter rather than longer.

All of these facts demonstrated the necessity of convincing the legislature to "make inquiries as to the state of health and value of life in all parts of the state, to ascertain where, and amidst what circumstances, most reach to the maturity of active being, where most sustain their strength to the full period, and where old age is most frequent and the latest postponed." Once the probable causes of life and death and health and disease were ascertained, the way would be open for future legislatures "to act for the better protection of the health and preservation of the life of the people." Jarvis, nevertheless, was quick to qualify his seeming support for an active and interventionist government. The public good, he noted, required the establishment of "negative principles of legislation, which grants no power, and enacts no law, that may create such conditions of things as will, in the least degree, and in the remotest time, affect the health of the people unfavorably." If the government gave permission to build a dam, for example, it would also have to provide protection for the health and lives of those who were adversely affected by the ensuing environmental changes. Positive government action, on the other hand, was a quite different matter. Conceding that English sanitarians favored regulatory legislation in regard to housing, pure air and water, drainage, and sewers, Jarvis proposed nothing definite in this matter. Nevertheless, just as the legislature encouraged agriculture, so it might offer rewards for plans dealing with housing, ventilation, heating, and draining stagnant waters and wetlands that sent forth "fogs, miasmata, and noxious effluvia." By authorizing a sanitary survey, Massachusetts would follow in the tradition of enlightened European nations and contribute toward the diminution of suffering, the creation of a healthier and more productive life, and ultimately the fostering of wisdom.[21]

The breadth of Jarvis's proposal proved too ambitious for most members of the general court. While sympathetic, they were not yet prepared to authorize such a survey. Instead they voted to print a large edition of the memorial and hold the matter over for consideration at the next session. Disappointed with the initial reaction, Jarvis set to work to build support for the project. He convinced the Massachusetts Medical Society to aid his efforts, and in January 1849 the society presented its own petition to the legislature which repeated most of Jarvis's arguments in favor of such a study. If anything, the society emphasized even more than Jarvis the economic benefits accruing to the community from improved health—an argument that was not lost upon legislators in a state where industry had become dominant. Moreover, the society was far less reluctant to endorse positive governmental action, insisting that it was indeed the legitimate business of government "to look after the interests of the people, and to watch, and protect, and encourage every thing that concerns the prosperity and happiness of the citizens of the State."[22]

While seeking legislative approval for the survey, Jarvis found time to prepare a lengthy article on English sanitary reform. Convinced that disease was not inevitable, he sought to persuade his fellow physicians that a broad environmental transformation could alleviate the immense suffering and degradation of the downtrodden urban masses. Summarizing the findings of Chadwick and the Health of Towns Association (founded in 1844 by Southwood Smith), Jarvis marshalled a mass of evidence to demonstrate that the shortened longevity and general debility of English workers were due to substandard housing, crowding, poor ventilation, nonexistent sanitary facilities, and impure water. There was also "a natural and habitual connection between filth and moral pollution, and also between outward neatness and inward purity."

But if suffering and misery had an environmental origin, then intelligent action could remedy this grave state of affairs. Jarvis was not hopeful that the urban poor could improve themselves, if only because they had never known anything but the environment into which they were born.

> When men and women have been accustomed from birth to no better condition, and no greater enjoyment, they marry and raise up children in the same privation and insensibility. They have no hope, and almost no desire, to leave their children in better condition than they themselves have endured.
>
> It is all in vain to expect, that improvement will arise out of the wants of those that need them most, that these people will either feel the desire and demand a better condition of things, or that they will have the moral or physical power to obtain it. . . .

The poverty of the poor includes more than a mere want of worldly substance. They suffer from want of health and physical strength, from defect of intelligence, of education, and of mental discipline, and from want of encouragement of their associates to improve their condition, and from lack of ambition to elevate themselves, and taste to enjoy more comfortable and more agreeable circumstances.

Their low physical, moral and mental condition prevents their acquiring property which come to those who have higher health and more mental energy; and their external poverty deprives them of the means of health and education. Personal character and power are intimately connected with outward prosperity and adversity. The poverty of the poor and the wealth of the prosperous are self-sustaining.

Leadership in the crusade to improve the lot of the urban poor, Jarvis concluded, would have to come from "the philanthropist, the political economist, and the legislative authority." This enlightened elite had a dual task. First, they had to transform the external condition of the poor by introducing needed sanitary measures to make urban environments healthier and more hospitable places. More importantly, the "education of the people" had to coincide with the "draining of streets and purification of houses." Jarvis closed his article with a warning calculated to build support for a sanitary survey. Noting that he had chosen English and European cities for analysis, he hinted that American cities could easily follow along a similar path unless preventive and remedial measures were adopted.[23]

The environmental transformation sought by Jarvis as well as other sanitarians was relatively limited in scope. They did not seek radical changes in existing economic relationships; their commitment to the sanctity of private property remained unyielding. Indeed, the appeal for change rested as much on the implied danger to the health of the entire community as it did on the necessity of fulfilling a religious imperative to uplift the poor. Disease, after all, was not especially selective, and there was no guarantee that even the righteous and clean would be able to avoid the epidemics that rapidly spread beyond their immediate point of origin.

Jarvis's discussion of the relationship between disease, environment, and morality also mirrored one of the fundamental dilemmas of mid-nineteenth-century medicine; namely, whether disease arose from deficiencies in personal character or from the nature of the environment and the social position occupied by the individual. Like others, Jarvis tended to move between both of these extremes and often to adopt positions inconsistent with earlier statements. The reason was not that he was insensitive to the issue, but rather that neither he nor any of his contemporaries could resolve two fundamental difficulties. First, the state of medical and scientific knowledge and technology made it virtually impossible to demonstrate a specific etiology. Before the specific germ theory of disease, etiological concepts tended to be either speculative or statistical in character; there was no way of establishing with any degree of certainty a relationship between a causative agent and a given disease. Secondly, the concept of heredity at this time was extraordinarily fluid in content. Laymen and physicians, as Charles E. Rosenberg has emphasized, assumed that acquired characteristics were inherited; that heredity was a dynamic process that did not involve fixed mathematical relationships; and that inherited qualities were general and protean rather than specific in nature (e.g., character and predisposition as contrasted with color of eyes or hair).[24]

The absence of a demonstrable etiology and a general theory of heredity susceptible to proof created obvious problems for physicians like Jarvis, problems that were never clearly recognized because of the absence of any means of satisfactorily resolving them. If, for example, disease was a function of individual behavior, *and* acquired traits could be inherited, could not an altered social environment change character and therefore behavior? The result of this intellectual and scientific dilemma was a debate marked by a peculiar inconsistency that reflected the puzzles posed by differential disease rates. Jarvis's discussion of this problem mirrored an ambiguity that could not have been resolved at that time, given the state of medical knowledge and the absence of a technology capable of facilitating a reorientation of basic etiological theory (the same holds true at present, although in a quite different form). Consequently, he vacillated between a concept of disease that at times placed responsibility upon individuals and at other times on the social and physical environment. His ambiguity would emerge even more clearly in his subsequent studies of high rates of mental and physical disease among Irish immigrants.

In May 1849 Jarvis's efforts bore results, for the legislature approved the appointment of a three-member commission to conduct a sanitary survey of the state. The election of Shattuck to the legislature undoubtedly aided the measure's passage, as did fear that the cholera epidemic would shortly be transmitted from Europe to the United States, where it would find a breeding ground among the poor and dissolute. The growing heterogeneity of the state's population also created a climate in which fear of alien immigrants, particularly the Irish, played a significant role. By 1845, as Shattuck had shown in his census of Boston, no less than one-third of that city's population of 114,000 was foreign born. To many Bay State residents their beloved commonwealth was confronted with the enigmas of slums, pauperism, disease, and crime. Since the Irish, more so than any other group, were associated with these developments, they bore the major share of the blame for the destruction of the beauty and homogeneity of the community as well as for rising tax bills that accompanied the increase in poverty and dependency. Still others feared the competition of Irish laborers willing to work for low wages. Above all, especially as the newcomers developed a sense of group consciousness, native perceptions of group differences increased markedly. Slowly but surely the older tradition of anti-Catholicism merged with the more recent fear of the changes that were transforming Massachusetts, giving rise to strong feelings of distrust and even hatred.[25]

In July Governor George N. Briggs appointed Shattuck, Nathaniel P. Banks, Jr., and Jehiel Abbott to the sanitary commission. Since the latter two lacked experience and knowledge, they were more than satisfied to delegate the job to Shattuck, who several months before had prepared an extensive report on the state's registration system for the legislature.[26] Within nine months Shattuck had completed and presented to the general court a report of more than five hundred printed pages. "We believe," he told the legislature in words that epitomized the sanitary movement, *"that the conditions of perfect health, either public or personal, are seldom or never attained, though* attainable.'' Throughout the Commonwealth evidence of deteriorating health was mounting as the salubrious environment that hitherto had fostered health was transformed by urbanization, immigration, and economic development. Citing a mass of statistical data, Shattuck detailed the extent of disease and mortality by age, ethnic, and occupational distribution of the population. In his view the evidence provided conclusive proof that the foreign-born had to bear a major share of the responsibility for the deterioration in health and the intensification of social problems. As immigration had increased, Massachusetts had resolved itself ''into a vast charitable association.'' Its medical, penal, and welfare institutions were inundated with hordes of foreigners, placing an excessive burden upon the state's taxpayers. ''The doors of these great institutions,'' he charged, ''have been thrown wide open; the managers of the pauperhouses of the old world, and the mercenary ship-owners who ply their craft across the Atlantic and pour their freight freely in, each smile at the open-handed, but lax system of generosity which governs us, and rejoice at an opportunity to get rid of a burden.''

But there was a still greater calamity attending to what Shattuck called ''this monstrous evil.'' Native residents who came into contact with immigrants became contaminated; their physical and moral powers deteriorated; and the ''healthy, social and moral character'' was forever lost. ''Pauperism, crime, disease and death,'' he warned, ''stare us in the face.'' To deal with such pressing threats, Shattuck offered a series of wide-ranging proposals, including more systematic efforts to ensure accurate data and the establishment of a decennial state census. His most important suggestion involved the creation of a general board of health to act as an adviser to the legislature in health-related matters. Whereas in the past he had been reluctant to support an active and interventionist government, he was now prepared to accept state responsibility for identifying problems and developing appropriate policies to deal with them.[27]

Initially Shattuck asked Jarvis to devise a plan for the survey and even to write the report. Jarvis declined both requests. His relationship with Shattuck had never been close. Each may have viewed the other as a rival, for Jarvis's ascendency within the

American Statistical Association was accompanied by Shattuck's eclipse. Jarvis may have also expected an appointment to the commission, for he had been instrumental in bringing about its creation. Whatever the reasons, Jarvis was reluctant to become involved in its operation. When Shattuck asked the Massachusetts Medical Society for advice, John C. Warren sent his letter to Jarvis with a request to prepare an answer. Again Jarvis declined, but did prepare a long communication in the name of the Society's counsellors, urging the commission to enumerate the hygienic resources and influences of the state, to reveal "the amount of vitality . . . life and health" enjoyed by its people, and to inquire into the differences, if any, in regard to life and health among residents. Jarvis, however, did meet frequently with Shattuck as the work of the commission progressed. Although the two had few disagreements on the necessity and importance of accurate statistics, they probably differed over some of the specific proposals contained in the final version.[28]

In January 1851 Shattuck's report was printed and two thousand copies were widely distributed. Shortly thereafter Jarvis published two reviews, the first of which appeared in the *Boston Medical and Surgical Journal*. At the outset Jarvis made clear his conviction that the commission had gone too far too fast. The original proposal for a sanitary survey, he noted, was limited to the gathering of data designed to show variations in health and longevity among different people in various locations. Out of such a survey would *ultimately* emerge measures designed to remove evils, protect life and health, and to enhance the state's sanitary condition. The initial request, therefore, was limited to the creation of a survey, for its supporters "thought not only that this was all that the Legislature and people were then prepared to undertake, but that, out of the information thus obtained reasons and arguments would be found for an efficient plan of removing and preventing the evils would be discovered." The commission, however, rejected gradualism "and have entered at once into all the length and breadth of sanitary organization and reform, and propose that the people grasp the whole matter in the beginning, and put it immediately into operation."

Jarvis then proceeded to summarize Shattuck's recommendations, which included repeal of all existing health laws in favor of a new modernized code; the establishment of a state board of health and local boards, all staffed by men of character, talent, learning, and tact; and the appointment of a secretary to the state board who would be the principal executive officer. The plan, he noted, resembled in some respects the successful arrangement adopted by the state for the supervision of its common schools; the state board of education had general supervisory authority while local committees implemented policy and presided over the schools in their local jurisdictions. Jarvis gave strong support to the proposal that all new towns and villages be compelled to adhere to zoning standards that ensured adequate light, air, water, drainage, and sewers. In this way the high mortality characteristic of densely populated urban areas would be reduced. The article closed by commending the report "to the careful consideration of the legislature and the people."[29]

In a much longer review in the *American Journal of the Medical Sciences* Jarvis repeated his previous summary and singled out for commendation the proposals that a uniform nomenclature for the causes of disease and death be adopted nationally to provide comparability and aggregation of data; that local sanitary associations be established in every town and city in order to educate the public; and that physicians emphasize much more than they had in the past their role in prevention of disease. He also quoted Shattuck's unfavorable portrait of the Irish, but indicated that the reasons for their poor health and weakened intellectual and moral powers had yet to be determined by the evidence. Although endorsing the commission's report, Jarvis expressed the fear that it comprehended more than the friends of the measure originally proposed and more than the legislature would adopt.[30]

Because of his commitment to the cause of sanitary reform, Jarvis's reviews tended to be outwardly favorable. Nevertheless, he hinted that Shattuck had gone too far in urging such a sweeping expansion of the welfare and police functions of government. The world, he later remarked in a brief biographical sketch of Shattuck, "was not ready" for his plan.[31] Nor did Jarvis agree with all of Shattuck's proposals, many of which "would prove impracticable and useless" since they could not become operational "until the state and the people should be cultivated and have grown to it by many years of trial and experience."[32]

Jarvis's reaction was symbolic of some of the divisions within the young sanitarian movement. That both men identified disease partially in terms of ignorance, vice, and immorality is uncontrovertible; in this respect they echoed the dominant beliefs of their age.[33] That both saw cities as the breeding grounds for diseases of all varieties is also clear; Concord rather than Boston remained their normative standard. Shattuck, however, demonstrated little compassion for the poor and believed that poverty was no excuse for filthy surroundings or unhygienic personal practices. Indeed, he attributed the filth and degradation of urban areas to the immigrants themselves, and urged the exclusion of those who might not be self-supporting or were incapable of being assimilated.[34] Above all, he feared that native Americans might very well be contaminated by the newcomers, a point of view widely shared by nativist Americans in the antebellum decades. Consequently, he did not hesitate to recommend an extraordinary expansion of the state's police powers to deal with the problems that seemed to be threatening the very fabric of the social order. Shattuck was persuaded of the propriety of using government to transform the immoral urban environment and thereby produce moral and virtuous citizens.

Jarvis, on the other hand, tended to see these issues in a somewhat different light. While agreeing with Shattuck that disease and death was a function of individual misbehavior, he rejected the interventionist solution that made government the arbiter of human destiny. Force would do little to reform individuals; what was required was an inner regeneration that would promote voluntary compliance with natural law. In place of force Jarvis substituted education. In 1850 he retained sufficient confidence in man's essential rationality to believe that few human beings would act in a manner contrary to their self-interest. And who would deny that increases in health and longevity were appropriate social goals? So confident was Jarvis in the ability of human beings to act in ways consistent with their self-interest that he argued that knowledge of the importance of fresh air would ipso facto lead factory owners to ensure that the housing of employees met minimum ventilation standards. A higher level of personal health would maximize productivity, and both would contribute to the physical, moral, and economic betterment of society.[35]

Perceiving a harmonious universe, Jarvis rejected out of hand any concept of irreconcilable class, social, or political conflict. Such conflict was simply the product of ignorance and unreason. The application of statistical knowledge to human problems would give rise to rational administration, which in turn would end once and for all the needless but dangerous conflicts so characteristic of human history. In this sense Jarvis's commitment to statistics was itself a general social theory that offered to the American people the alluring prospect of a harmonious and just social order. And if facts spoke for themselves, there was no particular need to spell out the details of social theory. Moreover, a commitment to an objectivity that rested on a factual foundation made it possible to rationalize conflict by placing responsibility for its existence upon the ignorance, emotionalism, and unreason of others; it also justified Jarvis's desire to play a key role in formulating social policy.[36]

Whereas Shattuck emphasized fear, therefore, Jarvis emphasized hope. The former felt compelled to advocate compulsion; the latter, voluntary compliance based upon knowledge of self-interest. In a significant sense Jarvis reflected in part the perfectionist impulse that played an important role in the social and medical thought of antebellum America.[37] Nowhere were the differences between the two better illustrated than in Jarvis's paper, presented at the meetings of the American Medical Association in 1850, dealing with the sanitary condition of Massachusetts and New England. Shattuck's interventionist recommendations reflected a conviction that deteriorating patterns of health were due to urbanization and immigration. Jarvis, on the other hand, remained unconvinced that the quality of the available data lent itself to any definitive generalizations. The shortcomings of registration reports and the life tables of insurance companies were obvious. But beyond this, Jarvis found that certain beliefs were simply not confirmed by existing data. A comparison of New York and Massachusetts, for example, did not necessarily demonstrate the latter's superiority. The higher percentage of deaths from old age in the Bay State was due largely to variations in age distribution; New York's population was younger. Even more surprising was the fact that in New York zymotic diseases were dominant in rural areas, while in Massachusetts they prevailed in the city. While longevity was greater in the country than in the city, it was not at all clear whether those who survived childhood had a better chance of surviving to old age outside of urban areas. Similarly, Jarvis was not convinced that consumption was actually more lethal in cities; the statistics had to take other factors into consideration before any clear answer could be given. On the other hand, Jarvis found that differences between the health of socioeconomic groups confirmed Chadwick's findings. Poverty, ill health, and shortened longevity all accompanied a diminished vital force. In his conclusion Jarvis reaffirmed his belief that much remained to be discovered, but that the rewards justified the quest.[38]

In the short run Jarvis's belief that Shattuck's plans were too radical proved to be correct.[39] By the time Shattuck had formulated his comprehensive plan the Massachusetts political scene was increasingly divided by factional strife. Conflict between natives and immigrants, between urban and rural interests—to say nothing about the antislavery issue—all combined to make reform a political rather than a moral issue. Without a broad consensus, proposals intended to transform society by redeeming individual morality were doomed to defeat from the outset. A plan that also rested in part upon an unfavorable portrayal of immigrant and urban groups was not likely to receive overwhelming support, given the growing political power of both. Moreover, the majority of the medical profession were themselves either disinterested or ignorant of sanitary reform and its emphasis on prevention; neither seemed applicable to private practice. Its members were far more concerned with immediate issues than with changing society. Finally, the fact that sanitarians relied on social and statistical data and often appealed to men who lacked medical training made the movement all the more suspect in the eyes of orthodox practitioners.[40] For these reasons it would be nearly two decades before Shattuck's proposal for a state board of health became a reality.

IV

Committed to making vital statistics the foundation of continued medical progress, Jarvis did everything within his power to further the collection and dissemination of such materials. To create an awareness of the significance of statistics, he single-handedly undertook to ensure that published materials—including national and local censuses, annual institutional reports, registration reports, sanitary investigations, and other comparable documents—received the widest possible circulation. At that time there was no system to facilitate scientific and medical exchanges. Few institutions of higher learning were research-oriented, and the concept of the research library was yet to develop. While it is true that learned and scientific societies played an important part in the dissemination and exchange of knowledge, the organizational void remained imposing.

What Jarvis did was to make his home the central clearing house for the collection and distribution of documents, particularly those pertaining to vital statistics. He assiduously collected multiple copies of documentary materials, which he then forwarded to other co-workers. During the 1850s and 1860s he corresponded with virtually every prominent American, English, and European figure then working in the field of vital statistics. Aside from his contacts with John H. Griscom, Edward H. Barton, T.R. Beck, and Elisha Harris, Jarvis was in touch with Adolphe Quetelet in Belgium, A. Legoyt in France, William Farr in England, and G. Varrentrepp in Germany, to cite only a few of the more prominent names. All of these individuals shared a faith in empirical and statistical investigations of the characteristics and problems of various population groups, disease patterns, and social problems in general. Referring to themselves as statisticians, they were in reality the demographers, economists, sociologists, epidemiologists, and actuaries of their age. ''The carelessness & indifference on these important subjects is beyond comprehension," remarked Barton in passionate words that expressed a widely shared view.[41] In a lengthy review article Jarvis echoed Barton and spelled out the potential benefits of a universal registration system. Properly compiled and analyzed, registration reports

> will give to the world very many important facts, in respect to life and mortality. They will enable us to take the first step toward ascertaining the sanitary and morbidic influences of seasons, atmospheric conditions and localities, of employments, social conditions, circumstances, and habits of the people. They will open the way to the discovery of the causes of disease, and probably to the means and methods by which they may be modified, ameliorated, and perhaps extinguished.[42]

Convinced that geographical, state, and even national boundaries were irrelevant to the operation of natural law, Jarvis did not neglect or overlook any potential source of reliable information. Slowly but surely his statistical and sanitary reputation grew to the point where he was the recipient of a multiplicity of queries concerning the availability and reliability of data and the organization of public and private investigations about social issues. Concerned with the difficulty of procuring documentary materials from as many nations as possible, Jarvis did not hesitate to call upon American diplomats abroad or political figures like Charles Sumner for aid. Eventually the burden became so great that he enlisted the aid of Joseph Henry at the Smithsonian Institution, who agreed to use his office to facilitate exchanges of material.[43] Consequently, Jarvis's reputation as a statistician reached the point where he was one of the best-known members of a growing scientific and scholarly community.

5

Insanity, Dependency, and Social Policy

While urging states to create an efficient system to collect vital statistics, Jarvis retained his concern for the welfare of dependent groups such as the insane, the blind, the deaf, and the feebleminded. His hostility toward an interventionist model of government did not preclude the adoption of ameliorationist policies for dependent persons and groups. Nor did his failure to secure a hospital superintendency diminish his fascination with insanity or his concern with social policy. Indeed, his faith in the efficacy of vital statistics reinforced his interest in insanity, and he continued to collect and analyze data that would contribute to a better understanding of the disease and aid in policy formulation.

The decade of the 1850s was destined to be his most productive period. During these years he wrote a series of significant papers dealing with insanity. His famous *Report on Insanity and Idiocy in Massachusetts,* published in 1855, was perhaps the single most comprehensive and influential study of its type during the nineteenth century and had an impact upon public policy for decades to come. Moreover, Jarvis became involved with the education of the blind and idiotic, and also began a two-decade association with the federal census in an effort to make it a true instrument of policy. By the close of the decade his name was familiar in his own country and abroad; he had finally achieved the fame and recognition that he had sought since early manhood.

I

Upon his return from Kentucky, Jarvis found that his home state was confronting all of the social problems associated with rapid population growth, immigration, and urbanization. The initial response to these changes was ambiguous, for economic growth also appeared to be accompanied by higher morbidity and mortality rates and increases in crime and dependency. To many citizens traditional institutions and behavioral patterns appeared increasingly irrelevant. The spontaneous and informal manner in which rural areas and small villages and towns during the colonial period dealt with disease and dependency failed to operate as well or as efficiently in growing urban areas, where a high rate of geographical mobility tended to limit social cohesion and the efficacy of traditional means of dealing with distress.

During the first third of the nineteenth century Massachusetts slowly but surely moved to adopt new institutional forms to meet pressing social problems. By 1830 the general court had enacted legislation establishing the state's first mental hospital and school for the blind. A few years later it established a state board of education. The tendency to respond in institutional terms was evident in public welfare as well, for the number of public almshouses increased rapidly. Such ameliorative activities, however, generally reflected individual and group pressures; they did not grow out of systematic policy formulation and social planning, if only because few state legislatures were structured to undertake such activities. The tenure of members was often brief and a high proportion served only a single term. Consequently, the legislative process inhibited consideration of a comprehensive social policy. The relative lack of institutionalization gave rise to laws that reflected individual problems and immediate issues.

Nor did early and mid-nineteenth-century lawmakers rely heavily upon professional expertise and bureaucratic personnel. Although legislatures were somewhat aware of the need for data that would serve as the basis for policymaking, the personnel, procedures, and even theories of social planning were not available. The absence of broad theoretical models relating to public policy made it difficult to gather or to use empirical data in meaningful ways, and legislative decisions often reflected external factors or assumptions that were never questioned. Lack of theory and methodology led to policies that in the long run had results quite at variance with the goals envisaged in the passage of the original legislation.

The lack of legislative institutionalization and structural cohesion as well as the prebureaucratic nature of state and local governments provided individuals like Jarvis with the opportunity to influence policy decisions. Lawmakers frequently relied on the talents and knowledge of strong-willed and determined figures who were authorities on a particular subject. Many of the most influential studies of mid-nineteenth-century social problems, including Howe's analysis of idiocy and Jarvis's report on insanity, were done by private individuals. Since the presentation and analysis of data generally implied a specific course of action, it was not surprising that Jarvis and others could influence the decision-making process.

Although committed to a voluntaristic political ideology, Jarvis was not averse to endorsing a more interventionist role for government in regard to distressed groups such as the insane, idiotic, blind, or deaf. Humanitarian and economic considerations dictated that society assume responsibility in order to help them overcome their disabilities, realize their potential, become productive citizens, and end all traces of neglect and mistreatment.

Beginning in the 1840s and continuing in subsequent decades, Jarvis broadened the scope of his activities. Unlike many of his contemporaries, he avoided political involvement; he preferred to confine his activities to work that would elevate rather than divide humanity.[1] One manifestation of this feeling was the support he offered to Samuel Gridley Howe, whose efforts on behalf of the education of the handicapped were already legion.

As a result of his work with blind and deaf children, Howe became aware of the feebleminded. Finding it difficult to educate and to care for them in an institution devoted to the physically handicapped, he urged that a separate facility be constructed. In 1846 the Massachusetts legislature authorized the appointment of a three-member commission to inquire into the subject of idiocy. Howe was chosen as its chairman and ultimately prepared his famous report on idiocy, which was completed in early 1848. Idiocy, declared Howe, was neither an accident nor a special dispensation of Providence; it was created by children or parents who "so far violated the natural laws, so far marred the beautiful organism of the body, that it is an unfit instrument for the manifestation of the powers of the soul." Rejecting any pessimistic conclusions, he insisted that mental defectives could be educated and made partially, if not wholly, self-supporting and independent. The legislature responded to Howe's appeal and provided a three-year appropriation to establish on a trial basis what became known as the Massachusetts School for Idiotic and Feeble-Minded Youth.[2]

The report on idiocy struck a responsive chord in Jarvis's mind. He immediately prepared a long review article for the *American Journal of the Medical Sciences*.[3] Although favorably disposed, Jarvis by no means accepted all of Howe's ideas, particularly the phrenological contention that mental deficiency was a function of cerebral development. Jarvis denied that science had established such a relationship; only future research would prove or disprove such an allegation.

However, Jarvis agreed with Howe's optimistic claim that the mental condition of most idiots could be improved. The public would benefit if the cost of supporting such persons could be reduced by making them partially or fully self-supporting. More importantly, humanitarian considerations demanded that these unfortunates be given "some idea of responsible life, some means and power of self-sustenance, and some self-respect." Society had two alternatives; it could mitigate the evil by educating mentally defective persons, or it could attack the conditions that caused idiocy. Jarvis favored the first because the latter alternative was simply too complex and difficult and did not lend itself to specific policies. "It is far easier," he told his readers, "to teach these stupid idiots, even to create intellect where it does not seem to exist, than to reform the morals of men and women, whose habits or indulgences lead to idiocy in themselves, or in their children, or to impress upon the world the necessity of looking only to the interests of the next and future generations in their marriage contracts, and in the management of their own persons.''[4]

In the autumn of 1848 the new facility for the education of the feebleminded was established on the grounds of the Perkins Institution and Massachusetts Asylum for the Blind, of which Howe was also the superintendent. Jarvis was intimately involved with the new project from its very inception. For over three decades he served as its secretary and also as superintendent pro tem during Howe's frequent absences. Howe was so deeply committed to a variety of activities that he often failed to provide leadership and direction. Moreover, he insisted that the school remain part of or adjacent to his home even though the physical plant was inadequate for the tasks at hand. The low state of the school, observed Hervey B. Wilbur in 1867, was the result of its substandard quarters and the fact that it lacked a full-time superintendent.[5] In part Jarvis filled the void, since he was admirably equipped to handle the innumerable details of institutional life efficiently. He helped recruit the staff; he supervised the development of the school's physical plant; he maintained a close watch over the administrative routine; and he aided efforts to secure legislative appropriations. When Howe was absent Jarvis usually visited the institution three to five times each week. Indeed, after Howe's death the trustees recognized Jarvis's contribution by electing him as the school's second superintendent, although ill health made his nine-year tenure in office largely honorary in character.[6]

In addition, Jarvis was associated with Howe at the Perkins Institution and Massachusetts Asylum for the Blind. In 1848 he became physician for that institution and assumed the superintendency during Howe's absence.[7] To Jarvis the education of the mentally defective and the blind was in some respects analogous to the care and treatment of the insane. All of these dependent persons required nutritious diets, exercise, and a clean environment. On the other hand, his concept of institutionalization was not monolithic. Insane and idiotic cases had to be separated from the environment that produced their deficiencies and subjected to an orderly regimen that taught new behavioral patterns. Blind children, however, were to be separated from others of their age ''only as far as is necessary for the peculiar instruction suited to their wants." Indeed, in urban areas it was desirable to have such children reside at home and attend special schools.[8]

II

Committed to institutional care and treatment of the insane, Jarvis was not convinced that public policy was grounded on an adequate foundation or appreciation of reality. State hospitals had multiplied, but little attention had been given to the overall magnitude of the problem, the nature of patient populations, the relationship between environment and mental disease, and the administrative and economic structures of institutions or their proper geographical location. Seeking to combine activism and scholarly detachment, he began to collect and to analyze data dealing with insanity, and ultimately wrote a series of original studies.

During his research Jarvis first became concerned with the physical placement of hospitals. At that time it was common practice to build public institutions at or near the geographical center of a state under the assumption that such location would provide all residents with equal access. In analyzing virtually every published hospital report, Jarvis found this assumption to be unwarranted. Taking into account the place of residence of all patients and the total population by county and state, he demonstrated that areas adjacent to hospitals used institutional facilities to a far greater extent than more distant regions. The precise ratios differed from state to state, since local factors, including the relative ease and cheapness of travel, determined use.

Such findings, Jarvis noted, contradicted the popular belief that the establishment of one or two state hospitals, centrally located, was an appropriate public response. Moreover, most states compounded their difficulties by expanding the size of their hospitals as use outstripped capacity. A change in public policy, he concluded, was in order. Since hospitals served surrounding communities, the public would gain by having a larger number of relatively small hospitals located in areas not served by any facility and accessible by regular and inexpensive modes of travel. Large hospitals, by way of contrast, served only the immediate area and, more importantly, often defeated their therapeutic goals by making moral treatment difficult, if not impossible.[9]

No person before Jarvis had ever attempted to demonstrate the fallacious basis of state policy. To be sure, Ohio apportioned admissions on the basis of county population, but this had not resolved the difficulties arising out of differential usage. The significance of Jarvis's article received immediate recognition. The *American Journal of Insanity* reprinted his conclusions, and his findings were often cited when legislatures discussed hospital placement.[10] Indeed, the policy of dividing states into districts served by specific hospitals (which became the norm by the end of the nineteenth century) was a direct result of Jarvis's pioneering study of the relationship between distance and frequency of use.

Shortly after the publication of his article, Jarvis, much to his discomfiture, inadvertently became involved in the famous Webster-Parkman case. In late 1849 Dr. George Parkman disappeared after visiting Professor John White Webster at the Harvard Medical School. After the discovery of a dismembered body in his laboratory, Webster was indicted for murder, found guilty, and sentenced to death in one of America's most famous criminal trials. The trial was controversial, partly because of the circumstantial nature of the evidence, the prominent persons involved, the vigor of the prosecution, and what some regarded as the prejudicial charge by Judge Lemuel Shaw. In early July 1850 the executive committee on pardons began hearings. A few days earlier a local clergyman who visited Webster in jail produced a purported "confession."[11]

Upon reading the "confession," Jarvis immediately wrote to Dr. Luther V. Bell, the head of the McLean Asylum and a member of the council. Webster's confession raised serious questions about the state of mind of both the victim and murderer, for a possibility existed that both were temporarily deranged. Parkman, wrote Jarvis, had visited him a week before his tragic demise. Shortly thereafter Jarvis had spent an afternoon with Samuel Parkman, the victim's nephew, who asked whether his uncle had behaved strangely. Jarvis responded in the negative, and Parkman replied that the family thought "he has been somewhat insane lately." Moreover, continued Jarvis, it had been rumored that Webster once nearly killed a colleague in a fit of rage. If either of the parties were not in possession of his senses, then the event would have to be cast in an entirely new light. Jarvis therefore felt obligated to place these facts before the committee on pardons, which could seek further verification.[12]

On July 8 Jarvis was called to testify before the committee. After discussing whether death could follow a blow on the head, Jarvis repeated the substance of his conversation with Samuel Parkman, and also read a letter from another physician describing Webster's violent reaction some years earlier. That same evening Samuel Parkman issued a public statement denying that he had spoken with Jarvis about his uncle before his disappearance or had expressed "the opinion or made the remarks which he [Jarvis] attributes to me." Obviously stung by the implication that his story was false or inaccurate, Jarvis immediately wrote to Parkman recounting their meeting in great detail and pointing out that during the trial Parkman (who was ill) could not testify because a deposition in a capital case was inadmissible. Expressing deep sympathy for the Parkman family, Jarvis concluded that he would have no choice but to issue a public rejoinder. Before taking this step, however, Jarvis preferred to have a meeting with Parkman.[13]

On July 18 Jarvis all but retracted his earlier statement in a letter to the governor's council.[14] Unfortunately, the surviving evidence sheds no further light on Jarvis's apparent repudiation of his previous statements. What is especially striking was Jarvis's ability to recall minor details relating to the alleged conversation, as well as the availability of corroborating evidence from others to whom he repeated the substance of the conversation. It is possible, of course, that Jarvis misunderstood Parkman's statement, but the circumstances militate against this explanation. There is some evidence of collusion on the part of the authorities. On July 17 one of the members of the committee on pardons wrote to the attorney general that his colleagues would recommend that Webster be executed on August 30—a strange statement in view of the fact that the hearings did not end until

July 18.[15] Whatever the case, Jarvis's retraction ended Webster's chances for clemency, and by the end of the month the sentence was carried out.

Some months earlier Jarvis had been asked to prepare a paper on the comparative liability of males and females to insanity, which he delivered at the meeting of the Association of Medical Superintendents of American Institutions for the Insane in the spring of 1850. Although his eligibility was doubtful, he had been admitted to full membership in the association in 1849, a reflection no doubt of his growing reputation.[16] The growing interest in diseases that seemed to demonstrate sex-related differences was a reflection of those nineteenth-century economic and social forces that were altering traditional roles of men and women. The result was a growing and often heated debate that invariably focused on the anatomical and physiological characteristics of the sexes. Some traditionally minded men employed medical and biological arguments in the hope of preserving traditional sex roles. Curiously enough, Jarvis's analysis of insanity went in a quite different direction; his conclusions directly contradicted the conventional view that women, because of their biological makeup, were more prone to mental disease than males.

To test the validity of the hypothesis that there was a higher rate of insanity among women than men—a view shared by most authorities, including Pinel—Jarvis analyzed the reports of about 250 American, British, Irish, Belgian, and French hospitals, some covering a period of many years. These reports, adjusted for the distribution of each sex in the general population, showed a higher incidence of insanity among males than females. Moreover, males had lower curability rates and higher mortality rates. What could account for these differences? The answer was not physiological; Jarvis insisted that neither clinical nor experimental evidence supported the popular view that there were "structural or functional differences of brain of the two sexes."

Having rejected a physiological interpretation of male and female differences, Jarvis turned to an examination of the temperament, character, and position of male and female. "The temperament of females," he wrote, "is more ardent, and more frequently nervous than that of males. Women are more under the influence of the feelings and emotions, while men are more under the government of the intellect.'' Yet Jarvis strongly qualified this statement when he argued that men had ''stronger passions and more powerful appetites and propensities.'' Indeed, he remained ambiguous on this subject, for he neither defined temperament nor clarified his position on the respective importance of environmental and hereditarian factors. In this respect he was somewhat atypical, for he did not accept many of the popular stereotypes of female intellectual inferiority.

Ultimately Jarvis explained varying rates of insanity in terms of causal factors that produced the disease. Men and women, he pointed out, played dissimilar social roles and hence were subject to different pressures. Men were more exposed to sensual temptation and the drive for material rewards; women were more exposed to emotional factors. Masturbation, excessive mental action in business, study, and politics, disappointed ambition, and accidents created more insanity among men than women ''not because women can bear these disturbing causes better than men, but simply because they are less exposed to them.'' On the other hand, grief, disappointed affection, domestic trouble, and fright produced more insanity in the female than the male because the former was affected by them far more frequently. Generally speaking, concluded Jarvis, ''those causes of insanity which act upon males are more extensive and effective than those which act upon females, and therefore, within the periods covered by the reports . . . and in the countries from which these reports come, males are somewhat more liable to insanity than females. But this must vary with different nations, different periods of the world, and different habits of the people.''[17]

Immediately thereafter Jarvis began to analyze the incidence and causes of insanity. His fascination with this topic was not atypical; most psychiatrists were concerned by the problem of causation precisely because of its implications for prognosis and therapy. The question of etiology, however, invariably involved prior moral judgments about the attributes of normative individual and social environments, if only because of the impossibility of establishing etiology through any known scientific means. Consequently, the psychiatric profession reflected the broader social and cultural ambiguity toward the nature and value of material growth. The same individual who hailed material progress as a harbinger of a new age could simultaneously interpret the present in terms of decline and posit the superiority of nature and natural man. Indeed, most mid-nineteenth-century psychiatrists insisted that civilization brought in its wake a sharp increase in the incidence of mental illness—a view that owed much to literary and philosophical romanticism.[18]

Aware of the extensive literature on the subject, Jarvis once again eschewed speculation and developed an argument based upon available data. In a paper delivered before the Association of Medical Superintendents of American Institutions for the Insane in 1851 (and repeated as a lecture before the Norfolk District Medical Society), Jarvis spelled out his own views. Conceding that many authorities believed that the incidence of mental illness was increasing, he nevertheless insisted that it was impossible to determine whether insanity was in fact increasing, stationary, or diminishing. Reliable data from earlier periods were all but nonexistent, to say nothing about the defects of current censuses. Nor could a comparison of hospital populations over time give any definitive indication of the prevalence of mental disease, for the founding of such institutions invariably transformed community sentiment by making families aware of the benefits of treatment and hence stimulating hospitalization. Equally fallacious were efforts to compare the number of insane persons in different countries, since comparable circumstances did not exist.

The fact that the past shed no light upon the incidence of insanity, however, was not an occasion for pessimism. By examining the *causes* of mental disease and determining "whether the causes are more or less abundant, and act[ing] with more or less efficiency now than formerly," it was possible to see whether or not more or less lunacy was being produced. The question, therefore, had to be restated in a more qualified form. Those causes related to the "malignant and the evil passions, anger, hatred, jealousy, pride and violent temper" remained the same, affecting savage and modern society alike. Causes connected with religious fervor had diminished. The increase in mental labor and greater social and economic mobility, on the other hand, all heightened the chances of becoming insane. "Thus we see," concluded Jarvis, "that with advancing civilization, and especially in the present age and in our own country, there is a great development of activity of mind, and this is manifested in most of the employments." The threats to sanity would prevail until mankind learned "the nature and the limit of their mental faculties" and governed themselves accordingly. Insanity, therefore,

> is then a part of the price which we pay for civilization. The causes of the one increase with the developments and results of the other. This is not necessarily the case, but it is so now. The increase of knowledge, the improvement in the arts, the multiplication of comforts, the amelioration of manners, the growth of refinement, and the elevation of morals, do not of themselves disturb men's cerebral organs and create mental disorder. But with them some more opportunities and rewards for great and excessive mental action, more uncertain and hazardous employments, and consequently more disappointments, more means and provocations for sensual indulgence, more dangers of accidents and injuries, more groundless hopes, and more painful struggle to obtain that which is beyond reach, or to effect that which is impossible.[19]

The generally favorable reaction to his views on mental disease stimulated Jarvis to continue his studies of insanity.[20] After the Massachusetts legislature passed a resolution providing for the establishment of a commission to investigate the problems relating to insanity in the spring of 1854, the choice of Jarvis as the key member was completely understandable.

III

When the Worcester State Lunatic Hospital opened its doors in early 1833, Horace Mann, the individual mainly responsible for its founding, not only felt a sense of pride and satisfaction but also expressed optimism for the future. Despite Mann's hopes, the Worcester institution, though enjoying some extraordinary successes in its early days and helping to stimulate a national movement to build public hospitals, never fulfilled the hope that it would serve as a central repository for the state's insane population by curing and discharging patients, thereby providing room for new cases. In 1836 and 1843 the legislature provided expanded facilities at the hospital, and the average patient population rose from 107 in 1833 to 359 in 1846. Such rapid growth had unforseen consequences, for the hospital's therapeutic role was increasingly subordinated to its custodial functions.[21]

The opening of a second state hospital in Taunton in 1851 provided only temporary relief; within three years the number of patients exceeded the total capacity of the two institutions. Moreover, conditions at the Worcester hospital continued to deteriorate. In view of the complex policy issues involved, the Committee on Public Charitable Institutions in 1854 urged the legislature to appoint a three-member commission to conduct a broad study of mental illness in the state and to recommend a "general and uniform system." The stage was now set for what was probably the single most significant and comprehensive investigation of mental illness and public policy in nineteenth-century America.[22]

Shortly thereafter the governor appointed Levi Lincoln, Increase Sumner, and Jarvis to the commission. The choice of Lincoln and Sumner was not surprising; both men had long been active in public life, the former as governor. The selection of Jarvis, on the other hand, indicated acceptance of the idea that the formulation of public policy required a collaborative relationship between political leaders and individuals possessing some degree of specialized knowledge and competence. Indeed, the modus operandi of the commission reflected this trend, for Lincoln and Sumner agreed in advance that Jarvis would collect all of the raw data, analyze its significance, and prepare the final report, subject only to their approval.[23]

Because of his conviction that generalizations must follow rather than precede the collection of data, Jarvis decided that a complete state census of the insane was in order.[24] He undertook to identify every insane person by name as well as to determine nativity, sex, race, age, means of support, place of residence or confinement, prior record of hospitalization, and prognosis. This information was solicited by polling physicians; in localities without physicians an identical form was sent to the resident clergyman. In addition, the superintendents of all public and private hospitals and keepers of jails and houses of correction in Massachusetts were included in the survey, as were hospital officials in other states. With the cooperation of the Massachusetts Medical Society and the press, over 800 returns representing about 1,400 individuals were received.[25]

The response to Jarvis's inquiry varied. Most correspondents simply supplied data and offered neither advice nor analysis.[26] In general, the returns were not enlightening about attitudes toward insanity and the insane. Occasionally a correspondent expressed his feelings. "Very many of the foreign Irish population," one Boston physician wrote, "say one in ten, imported into this city for the last six years, are idiots, or at least no better. Three fourths of the remaining Irish importations, are *mono-maniacs,* being the *dupes* of *Catholic priests.* One half of the whole receive aid from charitable institutions, the City or State."[27] Such comments, however, were atypical; the overwhelming majority of the responses simply provided the information requested by Jarvis.

After receiving the questionnaires Jarvis then checked the name of every mentally ill and idiotic person to make certain that the final figures took into account any duplicate reporting by different correspondents. The result was undoubtedly the most reliable census of the insane ever taken in the United States. According to the final tabulations, there were 2,632 insane persons in Massachusetts in the autumn of 1854. Of this number, 1,522 were paupers (693 supported by the state and 829 by towns), while 1,110 were supported by their own resources or by their friends. Only 625 were foreign-born; 2,007 were natives. At the time 1,284 were either at home or in town or city poorhouses; 1,141 were in hospitals; and 207 were in county institutions, houses of correction, jails, and state alms-houses. Perhaps the most revealing aspect of the survey was the fact that the overwhelming majority of those polled believed that most mentally ill persons were incurable. Out of the total of 2,632 insane persons, only 435 were regarded as curable, while 2,018 were listed as chronic cases (the prognosis of 179 was not reported). There were also 1,087 idiots in the state; 417 of them were supported at public charge and only 44 were foreign-born.[28]

After presenting a town-by-town breakdown of the number of insane persons, Jarvis moved on to an extended discussion of the relationship between pauperism and insanity. "There is manifestly a much larger ratio of the insane among the poor, and especially among those who are paupers," he pointed out, "than among the independent and more prosperous classes." What were the essential ingredients of poverty? In Jarvis's view poverty was much more than an external circumstance. It was rather an "inward principle, enrooted deeply within the man, and running through all his elements . . . . Hence we find that, among those whom the world calls poor, there is less vital force, a lower tone of life, more ill health, more weakness, more early death, a diminished longevity." Nor was the association between poverty and insanity a statistical accident; both were traceable to the same source, namely, an "imperfectly organized brain and feeble mental constitution" which carried with it "inherent elements of poverty and insanity."²⁹

Having analyzed the relationship between poverty and mental disease, Jarvis moved on to a discussion of what he called the "foreign element." He began by noting the greater incidence of insanity among foreigners (one case for every 368 persons) than among natives (one case for every 445 persons). Equally significant was the fact that 93 percent of foreign lunatics were paupers, as compared with only 57 percent of the native-born. There were two possible explanations for this state of affairs. Either foreigners (and by foreigners Jarvis was alluding largely to the Irish) were more prone to insanity, or else they were ill-adapted to the physical and cultural conditions of American society. Jarvis implied that both possibilities were partly true. "There is good ground for supposing," he wrote,

> that the habits and condition and character of the Irish poor in this country operate more unfavorably upon their mental health, and hence produce a larger number of the insane in ratio of their numbers than is found among the native poor. Being in a strange land and among strange men and things, meeting with customs and surrounded by circumstances widely different from all their previous experience, ignorant of the precise state of affairs here, and wanting education and flexibility by which they could adapt themselves to their new and unwonted position, they necessarily form

many impracticable purposes, and endeavor to accomplish them by unfitting means. Of course disappointment frequently follows their plans. Their lives are filled with doubt, and harrowing anxiety troubles them, and they are involved in frequent mental, and probably physical, suffering.

The Irish laborers have less sensibility and fewer wants to be gratified than the Americans, and yet they more commonly fail to supply them. They have also a greater irritability; they are more readily disturbed when they find themselves at variance with the circumstances about them, and less easily reconciled to difficulties they cannot overcome.

Unquestionably much of their insanity is due to their intemperance, to which the Irish seem to be peculiarly prone, and much to that exaltation which comes from increased prosperity.[30]

Although Jarvis seemed to establish a statistical relationship between insanity and pauperism, he had in reality made a far more fundamental point. What he had shown, at least to his own satisfaction, was that mental illness was greatest among the impoverished classes (which included a high proportion of Irish immigrants). Especially notable was the way in which Jarvis's prior assumptions conditioned his statistical methodology and the manner in which he established categories and then collected data. Jarvis began with the belief that poverty and ethnicity were the most significant variables; his data were organized accordingly. He did not, by way of contrast, consider the possibility that other variables (age, density of population, etc.) might be equally or more significant; hence his analysis all but ignored these factors. Although his questionnaire included information on age, for example, he did nothing with this material; in his eyes age played little or no role. Nor did he consider the possibility that sharp differences in the age distribution of immigrant and native-born populations might have explained (or narrowed) the glaring differential in their respective rates of insanity. Indeed, Jarvis was so committed to an explanation based on the primacy of poverty and ethnicity that on occasion he ignored a class mean that did not support his explanation. It must be kept in mind that at the time Jarvis prepared his report, the only statistical tool available to him was the class (or gross) mean. Neither adjusted means nor correlation techniques had yet been developed. Nevertheless, what remains impressive was the degree to which his use of particular class means was conditioned by prior beliefs; equally significant were the class means that he either ignored or else did not even aggregate. The survey of all institutionalized patients within Massachusetts revealed that when superintendents were asked about the prognosis of *individual* patients, their responses did not demonstrate the existence of differential curability rates. Of 705 natives, 127 (18 percent) were listed as curable and 578 (82 percent) as incurable; for 436 foreign-born the comparable figures were 79 (18.1 percent) and 357 (81.9 percent). These results, of course, did not confirm the relatively unfavorable portrait of Irish patients.[31]

Undoubtedly Jarvis was subtly influenced by the ethnic and economic conflicts of his age.[32] As tensions in the Bay State became more acute following the increase of Irish immigration, the attitudes of many social activists began to change. By identifying mental disease with poverty and ethnicity, Jarvis inadvertently supplied ammunition to groups that were beginning to question democratic and egalitarian assumptions. Within a generation some members of the New England intelligentsia would begin to agitate for an end to unrestricted immigration on the grounds that the superiority of the native stock was being threatened by the influx of inferior groups. In 1855, however, Jarvis stood midway between the faith of his youth and the fears that were to become more prevalent during the latter half of the nineteenth century.[33] The *Report on Insanity* reflected Jarvis's ambivalent attitudes; it was capable of being used for a variety of different purposes.

To Jarvis the most tragic part of the situation was that aliens were enjoying the advantages of state hospitals to a much greater extent than natives. Virtually every foreign insane pauper, he noted, was sent to a public institution, while only 42.7 percent of native paupers were institutionalized. Such a state of affairs, if unwise, was understandable. The bulk of the alien pauper insane, having no legal residence, were wards of the state; hence they were usually cared for in state-supported institutions. "Whatever may have been the design and the theory," Jarvis concluded, "the practical operation of our system is, to give up our hospital accommodations for permanent residence without measure to almost the whole of the lunatic strangers, while these blessings are offered with a sparing economy to a little more than a third of our own children who are in a similar situation.''[34]

Having dealt with both the extent of insanity and some of the social and economic factors involved, Jarvis moved on to a discussion of public policy. He began with the familiar proposition that it was more economical to incur the initial high costs of hospitalization and treatment than to support an insane person perpetually at a lower figure. One of the major problems confronting the state, however, was the narrow and shortsighted attitude of many localities, which preferred to incarcerate paupers in jails and almshouses instead of sending them to state institutions. Such a policy, he argued, was actually more expensive. The only alternative was to have the state assume greater responsibility for care and treatment. Not only should the Commonwealth provide additional hospital space, but it should compel its use by localities. Existing facilities, added Jarvis, were insufficient; on the basis of the accumulated data he concluded that there were about 700 more patients than there were places for them.[35]

After determining that a need for new accommodations existed, Jarvis wrote to a number of experienced psychiatrists for advice.[36] After evaluating their responses, he proceeded to discuss the basis on which policy ought to rest. Jarvis began with a favorable discussion of the recommendation of the Association of Medical Superintendents of American Institutions for the Insane that no hospital should have more than 250 patients.[37] Large hospitals diminished the effectiveness of moral treatment. He also insisted that a system of large hospitals scattered throughout the state was inferior to a system of more numerous but smaller hospitals, for any institution, regardless of size, tended to serve its adjacent area to a disproportionate degree. Jarvis's first major recommendation, therefore, involved the establishment of numerous small hospitals (250 patients or less) located in varying geographical areas.[38]

Next Jarvis considered the nature and characteristics of the patient population at an ideal hospital. Conceding that most of his correspondents favored separate hospitals for male and female, he was inclined to disregard this suggestion. A hospital of 250 for a single sex would have to draw its inmates from a wider geographical area, thus bringing into operation the generalization that areas distant from the hospital would use it the least. Similarly, he opposed separate establishments for curable and incurable patients. Not only was it difficult to determine whether or not a patient was incurable, but the mixture of both types in a single institution was mutually beneficial. Quiet demented patients had a soothing influence on the violent ones, and curable patients imparted hope to those less fortunate than themselves.[39]

On the other hand, Jarvis insisted that the hospital maintain the same social distinctions that existed in society at large. Indiscriminately mixing patients from all walks of life ran counter to human nature, and would also hinder the efficacy of therapy. While favoring retention of internal distinctions based on economic, social, and educational considerations, Jarvis opposed separate hospitals for native-born independent and pauper patients. Since there was an imperceptible gradation from the upper to the lower classes, it would be difficult, if not impossible, to draw fine distinctions between individuals who shared a basically similar way of life, regardless of their economic status. Cognizant of the British practice of segregating pauper from paying patients in different institutions, he pointed out that the English poor were ignorant and uncultivated, and that a much wider gulf between classes existed there than in the United States. Under these circumstances the English authorities were justified in discriminating between patients on the basis of class.[40]

Jarvis, however, included one significant exception to his recommendation that independent and pauper patients be admitted to the same institution. Specifically, he argued that state paupers (those who had no legal residence in Massachusetts)—most of whom were Irish aliens—could not be classified in the same category as native paupers. Coming from a different environment and holding dissimilar customs, attitudes, and religious beliefs, these aliens resembled the English poor rather than the native poor. The interests of all would best be served by keeping native and alien paupers apart. In this way the latter could be kept in institutions that recreated a "style of life" not very different from the one to which they were normally accustomed. Such a policy had the added virtue of economy; institutions that cared for the alien pauper insane could be maintained at a lower cost than those caring for native patients, since the former required fewer amenities than the latter. Jarvis, in addition, suggested that institutions for the alien pauper insane provide separate quarters for criminal lunatics.[41]

Having discussed the problems of mental disease, Jarvis and his fellow commissioners then offered five distinct proposals to improve conditions and to establish a consistent policy for the Commonwealth. First, they urged that a new hospital be built, preferably in the western part of the state. Second, the sale of the Worcester hospital should be postponed until the new one was ready for occupancy. Third, the legislature should consider the possibility of establishing a separate hospital for state paupers. Fourth, the law of 1836, which required counties to maintain institutions for the nonviolent insane, should be repealed and the counties thereby relieved of responsibility for these persons. Finally, the laws relating to insanity and hospitals should be revised and a more modern and systematic code be adopted.[42]

Early in March 1855 the final report was sent to the legislature. So thoroughly had Jarvis done his work that few critical or dissenting voices were heard. On the contrary, the initial reception of the report was favorable. The Committee on Public Charitable Institutions arranged for 10,000 copies to be printed (in place of the normal edition of 1,600) and distributed locally and nationally; it also asked Jarvis to draft its report to the full legislature and the law providing for the establishment of a new hospital. When the bill came up in the legislature it encountered little opposition; in less than three months a hospital for 250 patients and an appropriation of $200,000 had been authorized.[43]

The immediate result of Jarvis's work was the decision to erect a new state hospital in Northampton, thereby giving the western part of the state access to a public facility. Jarvis's role gained immediate recognition, for he was invited to give the address at the laying of the hospital's cornerstone.[44] On the other hand, he was not selected as a member of the building committee, a fact that he attributed to the practice of offering such positions to local political figures. Nevertheless, Jarvis remained involved in the hospital's progress, especially after the legislature's favorable attitude began to change and sentiment for discontinuing the project grew; he immediately began to rally support. After considerable acrimony the Northampton hospital was completed in 1858.[45] Ironically, Jarvis once again failed to be selected as its first superintendent, a position he coveted and one that momentarily seemed to be within his grasp.[46]

If the sole result of the *Report on Insanity* was the erection of a single additional state hospital, it would hardly have merited Jarvis's own judgment that the project was "the most successful of his life."[47] Far more significant were the long-range and intangible results of his study, which easily transcended the founding of another public institution. Aside from the statistical data and the recommendations that the state assume greater responsibility for the mentally ill, Jarvis's most important contribution was his discussion of insanity in terms of class, ethnic, and social differences. In this respect he helped to pave the way for the discussion of social problems generally in such terms; his analysis anticipated the future evolution of the social and behavioral sciences and the growing reliance upon "scientific" social surveys to illuminate pressing problems. Although the report itself was couched in measured and qualified terms, it could be used by others much less concerned with accuracy and in ways that Jarvis would not have approved.

Far more than any individual before him, Jarvis had explicitly related poverty to insanity and offered hard data to prove his case. In the long run, therefore, he inadvertently supported the growing belief among many Americans that poverty and character were related and that mental (as well as other) diseases were associated with impoverished groups, particularly those coming from a minority ethnic background. His data, moreover, seemed to show an extraordinarily large number of incurable cases (although Jarvis himself strongly reiterated his conviction that mental disease, given early treatment, was a largely curable malady). The result was that the *Report on Insanity* reinforced an unfavorable image of state hospitals. For if state institutions received predominantly lower-class patients (as indeed they did) whose illness was related to moral deficiencies, did it not follow that they were undesirable (although necessary) places, especially if alternatives were available in the form of private asylums that accepted a more restricted clientele?

Also notable was the fact that Jarvis did not think it necessary to defend the validity of institutional care and treatment of insanity; in his eyes institutionalization was an assumption rather than a proposal that required justification. By this time the treatment of insanity within a hospital was the norm; neglect or incarceration in welfare and penal institutions was abnormal. This is not to imply, as some critics have argued, that an institutional response to distress represented a narrowing of the moral parameters of the community or a conscious effort to impose a pattern of social control on nonconformist behavior (especially if such behavior was associated with lower-class groups).[48] To Jarvis such an allegation would have seemed totally alien. All behavior, he maintained, had an organic concommitant; it therefore followed that abnormal behavior was associated with a somatic abnormality. Given his belief that the very existence of society presupposed objective behavioral standards, it was natural for him to support institutional care and treatment not simply to protect the community, but to aid distressed persons.

IV

Had the *Report on Insanity* been merely another parochial document of concern only to the residents of a single state, it would hardly merit a prominent position in the social history of American psychiatry and welfare in the nineteenth century. Many other state and local studies of mental illness, after all, have been consigned—with good reason—to virtual oblivion. The *Report on Insanity,* however, occupies a somewhat unique place in the history of public policy toward mental illness. It stands apart from other comparable investigations if only for the wealth of detail and the effort that went into its preparation. But in addition, its analysis and conclusions anticipated the future evolution of mental hospitals, although in a way not clearly perceived by Jarvis and his contemporaries. Having introduced class, ethnic, and social factors into his discussion of public policy, Jarvis never realized (nor was there any reason why he should) that these would far outweigh his prevailing optimism about the prognosis of mental illness. In the long run, there-fore, his study reinforced public antipathy, especially after men-tal hospitals assumed the responsibility of providing custodial care for poor and indigent groups.

The significance of the *Report on Insanity* was further enhanced by the influential role of the Commonwealth of Mas-sachusetts during the nineteenth century. Aside from the literary and intellectual reputation of some of its residents, the Bay State was also a leader in developing institutions and struc-tures relating to welfare and philanthropy, to say nothing of its activities in education. It was the first state to develop a compre-hensive system of public mental hospitals; it pioneered in the field of public health; it also established the first Board of State Charities—the forerunner of the modern state welfare depart-ment. Other states tended to emulate its policies. As a result, the *Report on Insanity* received far greater notice than other comparable state studies of social and medical problems.

The relatively wide circulation of the report was due in part to Jarvis's own indefatigable efforts. He saw to it that copies were sent to every Bay State physician, to hospital superintendents at home and abroad, and to innumerable libraries. Joseph Henry at the Smithsonian provided aid in distributing the book abroad. The initial private reaction was positive. John S. Butler of the Hartford Retreat described the report as *"valuable* and a monument of rare industry as well as of ability''; he requested a dozen copies to use in Connecticut in efforts to improve condi-tions among the insane and idiotic. Butler's enthusiastic recep-tion was by no means atypical; most recipients of the volume thought that the data and policy proposals heralded a new era in care and treatment. The public reaction of psychiatrists (includ-ing Bell, Kirkbride, and Ray) was equally favorable. The Asso-ciation of Medical Superintendents of American Institutions for the Insane unanimously adopted a resolution characterizing Jar-vis's work ''as the first successful attempt, in America, to secure entirely reliable statistics on this subject'' and expressing gratifi-cation at the action of the legislature in approving a third state hospital.[49]

The laudatory comments by the leaders of the young psychiatric speciality were seconded by both the *Boston Medical and Surgical Journal* and the *American Journal of Insanity.* Reviews by individuals were equally favorable.[50] Pliny Earle thought the book significantly important to merit a detailed summary of its evidence and conclusions.[51] Earle's comments were echoed by an article in the *Journal of Prison Discipline and Philanthropy,* the organ of an influential group of Pennsylvania prison reformers. That the *Journal* emphasized Jarvis's discussion of pauperism was not surprising, since it had as one of its primary goals the extirpation of crime (which it related to poverty, indolence, and an imperfect welfare system). The thrust of this article demonstrated the peculiar relationship that some Americans drew from Jarvis's discussion of poverty and insanity—a relationship that played a crucial role in the evolution of the mental hospital.[52]

Undoubtedly the most detailed and perceptive analysis of the *Report on Insanity* was written by Isaac Ray and published in the *North American Review.* Possessed of a keen, inquiring, and skeptical mind, Ray's preeminent position in American psychiatry was established in 1838 when he published his classic work on the medical jurisprudence of insanity. Throughout his long career Ray subjected much of the accepted knowledge about mental disease to rigorous scrutiny and often found it wanting. His analysis of the Jarvis report, therefore, was that of an individual acknowledged as one of the foremost leaders in the specialty.[53]

Ray began his paper by pointing out that statistical evidence had hitherto been ambiguous in nature. The major contribution of the Jarvis report was its "accuracy, completeness, and pertinence." Nevertheless, he was not convinced that the report was entirely free from error. He agreed with Jarvis that the incidence of insanity in Massachusetts was higher than in other states, but insisted that Jarvis's explanation of this fact (namely, that the foreign insane were more numerous than the native-born insane as compared with the same population of their respective classes) did not necessarily follow. Ray particularly objected to the way in which the report dealt with idiocy, for he was not certain that adult idiots constituted a class distinct from the mentally ill. He also believed that non-psychiatrists lacked the expertise that was required to distinguish between idiocy and insanity. Moreover, if the total number of idiots (especially adults, who outnumbered idiots under the age of sixteen by three to one) were counted with the insane, the claim that the incidence of mental illness was highest among the foreign-born was invalid.

If the incidence of insanity in the Bay State could not be attributed to the accretion of immigrants in the population, what could account for it? The figures, Ray noted, did not lend themselves to the popular explanation that mental illness was more prevalent in manufacturing and mercantile communities than in farming areas. Indeed, some evidence indicated that older and more stable communities had the highest rates of insanity. Since at least one-third of all cases of insanity were due to heredity, areas with an inbred population tended to perpetuate and to increase the frequency of this malady. Nevertheless, Ray did not attempt to provide a definitive answer to the problem of the high incidence of insanity in the commonwealth.

Ray then moved on to a discussion of the relationship between poverty and mental illness. In this respect it is worth noting that virtually every analysis of the *Report on Insanity* sooner or later focused on Jarvis's discussion of this subject. Without doubt, argued Ray, insanity "may be traced, in many instances, more or less directly to poverty." After quoting Jarvis's statement that poverty was an "inward principle," he nevertheless questioned whether the kind of destitution implied in the report was particularly common in the United States. Yet in the next paragraph Ray expressed some doubt about the curability of insanity among foreigners as compared with native Americans. In New England hospitals Irish patients were "preeminently incurable, though promptly subjected to hospital treatment."[54] Moreover, there was no question but that the Irish occupied a disproportionately high percentage of places in hospitals and other receptacles. In discussing this state of affairs, Ray strongly supported the recommendation that the state establish a separate institution for foreign insane patients; natives and aliens alike would benefit from homogeneous grouping.

Ray then followed up his proposal for a separate institution for foreign insane paupers with a suggestion that the commonwealth consider the feasibility of establishing two hospitals for state paupers. The first would care for curable patients; the second would provide custodial care for incurable cases. The former would by necessity remain small, since the requirements of therapy were complex and demanding. The latter, on the other hand, could accept more cases, and subordinate staff could supervise much of the daily routine. Ray concluded his discussion by expressing the hope that Massachusetts would fully meet its obligations toward the insane.[55]

Jarvis's contemporaries were not far wrong in recognizing the nature of his achievement even though their perception of his influence would be far less accurate. In many respects the *Report on Insanity* was a model social survey for its age. Jarvis began with a monumental effort to identify all known insane persons, their vital statistics, and the types of facilities available. From these data emerged a series of generalizations, some of which reflected his own ideological perceptions, especially his prior assumption that behavior, environment, and disease were inseparably linked. Finally, he offered a series of specific proposals within a general policy framework. In this respect he anticipated the social surveys characteristic of twentieth-century social and behavioral science.

Yet Jarvis's hope for a more enlightened and humane future was in practice never fully or even partially realized. His analysis of the relationship between poverty and disease, as well as some of his other statistical generalizations, was capable of being used in quite different ways, particularly in times when social tensions were exacerbated by economic stress. Jarvis's portrait of the Irish, for example, was couched in relatively moderate terms. Yet his own data and words could lead to far more invidious conclusions. And his proposal to segregate native and immigrant patients only served to reinforce prevailing hostile stereotypes.[56]

Moreover, the incremental nature of the legislative decision-making process could—and did—easily transform Jarvis's recommendations by ignoring their general context. Thus the Massachusetts legislature acted favorably on his request for a third public hospital, but ignored the stipulation that its size be limited. Nor was there a long-range commitment to construct a series of small hospitals geographically distributed, thereby providing all areas with accessible facilities. The absence of the very concept of social planning inhibited any consideration of priorities, thereby reinforcing an incrementalism that often gave rise to results quite at variance with the objective of particular policies. Finally, legislators, for obvious reasons, were in no position to evaluate the analysis of their own commission, particularly when the findings and proposals appeared to represent professional authority. Consequently, a serious debate on existing or alternative policies and their respective costs was virtually absent.

V

Although the *Report on Insanity* represented by far Jarvis's most significant achievement, he was not content to rest upon his laurels. At the meetings of the Association of Medical Superintendents of American Institutions for the Insane in 1856 the members heard a paper prepared (but not delivered) by Jarvis dealing with the criminal insane. Prior to this time hospital superintendents generally ignored the question of psychiatric treatment for insane convicts, perhaps because they feared that the reputation of their institutions might suffer if it became known that convicted criminals were admitted as patients. Public policy, Jarvis noted, often confused criminals who became insane after their conviction with those who committed crimes while insane. The criminally insane (whom he designated as ''insane transgressors'') were guiltless, since they were not responsible for their actions. Conceding that both threatened public security and required restraint, Jarvis nevertheless insisted that the issue of their disposition was by no means resolved by existing practices. Indeed, insane criminals often received milder punishments by virtue of the fact that they were incarcerated for definite terms whereas the criminal insane were imprisoned for indefinite periods. The existing practice of confining both classes in prison was also objectionable. Insane criminals no longer comprehended the reasons for their imprisonment, while insane transgressors were punished for acts for which they were not legally responsible. Above all, prisons were incapable of providing the treatment to which all diseased individuals were entitled. If the ends of justice and humanity were to be served, a new policy was required. Neither insane criminals nor the criminally insane belonged in prison while their insanity continued. On the other hand, it was equally unjust to confine insane convicts in hospitals, thereby forcing "the high-minded and self-respecting to associate with the guilty and corrupt" and disrupting the administration of the hospital as well. Similarly, it was unfair to force the criminally insane to associate with individuals whose criminal activities had led to their imprisonment. Assuming that all had a right to treatment, Jarvis surveyed existing practices and found them wanting. The maintenance of a "hospital" within prison grounds was unacceptable, since it precluded a therapeutic environment or adequate occupational facilities. Ultimately Jarvis recommended that a separate hospital for insane criminals be established. The disposition of the criminally insane could then be left to the courts, which would have the option of sending them to a state hospital or the hospital for insane criminals. Recognizing that few states had a sufficient number of insane convicts to establish its own institution, Jarvis urged a policy of cooperation that involved the founding of one institution that served a number of states.[57]

While studying different aspects of public policy, Jarvis continued to support preventive measures. Hoping to reach a wider audience, he persuaded Henry Barnard, editor of the *American Journal of Education*, to publish in 1858 a paper dealing with education and insanity delivered some years earlier at the convention of hospital superintendents. In it Jarvis reiterated his belief that a proper education could do much to prevent mental illness.[58] A year later he repeated much the same theme in a lengthy contribution for the *North American Review*.[59] To Jarvis life remained a moral venture in which human beings perpetually struggled to maintain a proper balance between competing forces that threatened to disrupt their equilibrium. In this respect he never outgrew the influences of his youth and education. The resolution of social problems required the application of knowledge and an intelligence guided by a mature moral sense. Given effective use of these traits, it was possible to create an institutional structure that would help to reduce the burdens that dependency placed upon the individual and society. To this end Jarvis directed a large part of his energies during the 1850s.

6

The Federal Census

The *Report on Insanity* gave Jarvis more than satisfaction and recognition; it confirmed his conviction that social improvement was dependent upon accurate and comprehensive statistical data. Recognizing that the ability of individuals to gather such material was limited, he began to seek more systematic means of collecting aggregate data that would ensure accuracy, continuity, and comparability. The virtues of accuracy were self-evident. The need for continuity and comparability, on the other hand, was not as well recognized. Jarvis, therefore, wanted to find some means to guarantee that the collection of data would never cease, thereby minimizing the risk that generalizations would represent special rather than general cases. He also hoped that it would be possible to specify clear and universally acceptable classification systems, and thus make possible the discovery of scientific laws.

The decentralized nature of American society and government, however, seemed to pose an insuperable barrier to the fulfillment of his plans. Although some urban areas and states provided for mandatory registration of births, marriages, and deaths, the data collected were often incomplete or not organized within appropriate categories. Moreover, Jarvis's conception of data transcended the more limited objectives of registration; he envisioned statistics that illuminated the complex relationships between social structure, population, environment, and social problems. Ultimately he turned to the federal census. National in scope, the census possessed the potential to provide the raw materials required by scientific investigators and to ensure continuity and comparability, thus enhancing the utility of its data.

Yet Jarvis recognized that the census as then constituted could not achieve the scientific objectives he sought. It lacked a permanent structure; it was deeply influenced by partisan politics; it did not have a commitment to standards of honesty and integrity; and its staff lacked both scientific training and a vision of the potential significance of the data gathered. When in 1849 Jarvis received a letter soliciting his advice about the forthcoming census of 1850, he became involved in a twenty-year effort to alter the organization and design of the federal census in order to heighten its usefulness to the scientific community and to the elected representatives of the American people. During the 1850s he emerged as one of the single most influential advisers to the superintendent of the census. In the 1860s he was put in charge of preparing the mortality statistics. And in 1869 and 1870 he served as an adviser to Congressman James A. Garfield, who was then promoting legislation designed to eliminate some of the more glaring defects in the census.

I

Jarvis's growing interest in the potential importance of the census reflected his broader concern with social problems during the 1850s.[1] Ultimately he came to the conclusion that a revamped census was indispensable for medical and social research. In placing the census within this new (and radical) perspective, Jarvis joined a small but growing international community of scientists, physicians, and social researchers who shared his faith in the paramount importance of classification and collection of aggregate data. By this time several currents had converged to give rise to a type of social inquiry whose methodological distinctiveness was a commitment to quantitative research. The seventeenth-century mercantilist concern with population and vital statistics was reinforced by nineteenth-century Baconian science, which tended to identify all of science with taxonomy. To this was added the fascination with *social* problems characteristic of virtually all modernized nations in the West. This fascination, in turn, stimulated interest in quantitative methods to a degree where virtually all significant problems were defined and described in statistical terms. Underlying the application of a quantitative methodology was the assumption that such a methodology could illuminate and explain social phenomena. Consequently, early and mid-nineteenth-century science and medicine were preoccupied with the development of elaborate classification systems capable of ordering a seemingly infinite variety of facts.

The emphasis on quantitative research resulted in a rapid proliferation of statistical societies and social investigations during the first half of the nineteenth century. Indeed, the first International Statistical Congress, attended by individuals representing a significant number of national statistical associations, met in Brussels in 1853. Most statisticians, including Jarvis, shared a radical faith that quantitative research, when merged with administrative rationality, could replace politics; they took for granted that the nature and purpose of human society was defined by natural law. In their eyes statistical knowledge should determine social policy, and thus put an end to the pernicious bickering over theory, principles, and politics.

While many figures contributed to the development of quantified social research during the nineteenth century, Adolphe Quetelet was virtually unsurpassed in importance. Born in Belgium in 1796, Quetelet's most enduring and significant work was in his refinement of social statistics. Not only did he pioneer in establishing procedures to enhance the accuracy of national censuses, but he never tired of calling attention to the need for accuracy as well as uniformity and comparability of data. Consequently, he played a leading role in the organization of the International Statistical Congresses, which helped to establish communication between like-minded individuals from many Western nations.

Deterministic in his outlook, Quetelet maintained that statistical averages depended upon social conditions and varied with time and place. The implications of this position were monumental; it meant that causal factors could be isolated, since a change in social conditions would be followed by a change in averages. Paradoxically, Quetelet, like others of his generation, did not permit his commitment to determinism to inhibit his advocacy of consciously guided social change; he insisted that humanity had the power to improve its condition, for a change in social institutions would by definition alter the ensuing results.

Reliable generalizations, Quetelet reasoned, could only be obtained by the study of many rather than few individuals. Herein lay the true method for all valid social research. And what could be more important than accurate censuses, which would provide a large body of uniform and comparable data to illustrate social organization and social phenomena. Were these censuses taken at regular intervals and in different places, the result would be a body of material that would ultimately give rise to precise general propositions. Statistically speaking, Quetelet wanted to use these data to determine averages and the limits of variations. The ultimate goal was to measure in a quantitative manner the relationship of two or more variable elements throughout their distribution.

Yet Quetelet never moved beyond simple statistical averages; the discovery of the correlation coefficient had to await the work of Francis Galton and Karl Pearson at the end of the nineteenth century. Quetelet's goal was to concretize the "average man." As a result, he never recognized the importance of the distribution of deviations from the average; his method consisted largely of comparing averages in different populations. Deviations from typical means could only be due to accidental causes, which by definition could not be explained in a scientific manner. Because of Quetelet's influence, mid-nineteenth-century social statistics emphasized the collection of data and the comparisons of averages.[2]

Jarvis, like Quetelet, never grasped the significance of distributions of deviations from the mean. Hence he was also concerned primarily with the computation of averages. Given the simplicity of this statistical model, it was understandable that Jarvis would place as much emphasis upon the classification and collection of data as he would upon their systematic analysis. This is not in any way to suggest that he was disinterested in the use of data. It is only to say that prevailing statistical theory severely limited the *kind* of analysis that later became characteristic of modern social science.

Although his faith in statistics remained unshaken, Jarvis was troubled by the unreliability and paucity of raw data. Even the federal government refused to disclaim the errors in the sixth census. Nor was the census of 1850 an improvement over its predecessor. In some places, Jarvis wrote to Quetelet, fewer than half the deaths were reported, to say nothing about the gross exaggeration in the size of the foreign-born population.[3] Such imperfections, however, were no reason for pessimism. On the contrary, forceful and intelligent action could remedy the situation and bring into being a modernized census. Then, with the cooperative efforts of census takers in other countries, social research could be raised to a new level.[4]

If, as Jarvis maintained, science was based upon classification and the collection of aggregate data, then clearly the census was an indispensable instrument of research. Like many other contemporary scientists and physicians, Jarvis was somewhat oblivious to the philosophical difficulties of developing a taxonomy based upon the subjective perceptions of the observer, and also tended to identify the existence of a statistical relationship with causality. Nor did he realize that the classification of a fact was not the same as knowing the fact in a scientific sense. Consequently, he was able to make a formidable intellectual leap and see in the census a definitive means of classifying knowledge and articulating generalizations that would aid in the task of social regeneration. His religious and philosophical training, combined with his disillusionment with conventional medical therapies, inexorably led him in the direction of modern social research with its increasingly elaborate classification categories and its affinity for quantification.

II

As 1850 drew near, demands for the reform of the federal census increased, for by this time its shortcomings were well recognized. Aside from gross inaccuracies, earlier censuses were virtually limited to the enumeration of population, although those of 1810, 1820, and 1840 attempted, with little success, to extend the scope of the inquiry to include business and industrial statistics. One of the most formidable barriers to an accurate and comprehensive compilation was the absence of a permanent agency. Each decade a new but temporary office was created, staffed by political appointees and inexperienced clerks. Suggestions for the establishment of a permanent federal statistical bureau met with little success.[5]

In 1848 Congress began to study the forthcoming census. Some members were disposed simply to revive the schedules used in 1840. This proposal caused some consternation among statisticians, since it threatened to perpetuate earlier shortcomings. The American Statistical Association was already agitating for a restructuring of the census. One of its members, Senator John Davis of Massachusetts, served as a conduit in Congress for the views of those individuals concerned with more accurate and complete data. Early in 1849 Congress enacted legislation establishing a census board to prepare the forms and schedules for the new census. The board selected Joseph C. G. Kennedy, a Pennsylvania Whig, as its secretary. Kennedy immediately solicited the advice of such eminent figures as Shattuck, Archibald Russell of the American Geographical and Statistical Society, and Jarvis. In a long communication Jarvis offered a general plan for the taking of the census and a detailed analysis of the types of vital statistics that he hoped would emerge as the final product. Kennedy then drafted six schedules covering the free and slave populations, mortality, agriculture, manufacturing, and social statistics. These were eventually adopted, although not without conflict.[6]

The census of 1850 provided for a significant extension in the number and scope of categories. For the first time a separate schedule gave the name, age, sex, color, marital status, place of birth, occupation, and date and cause of death of every person who had died during the twelve months preceding June 1, 1850. The latter schedule was clearly the result of efforts of men like Shattuck and Jarvis, who were seeking the requisite national statistics to enable them to specify the precise environmental conditions that promoted health and disease. Equally significant, the process of planning the census involved leading social statisticians, thereby establishing a precedent. Indeed, when Kennedy solicited advice, Jarvis responded by warning that it was a matter of the highest importance to make certain that honest men were employed as census takers. In the past, he noted with regret, the census had been taken by politicians who were "in the habit of looking at facts as raw material to be altered, curtailed or expanded to suit an ulterior purpose."[7]

Between 1850 and 1853 (the period during which the census was being taken and the results totalled), Jarvis had no direct contact with anyone in Washington.[8] In early 1853 Kennedy was replaced by J.D.B. De Bow, the eminent Southern journalist whose magazine *(De Bow's Review)* championed Southern mercantile and agricultural interests, states' rights, and Southern nationalism.[9] Jarvis's first contact with the new superintendent came in the summer of 1853 when he sought access to some of the mortality data from the census office. Having examined some of the preliminary aggregate figures for the state of Maryland, Jarvis expressed disappointment with several schedules and noted that "some valuable element was omitted." Despite his reservations, he looked forward to receiving the final product in order "to compare our own condition with that of other nations as shown by their censuses."[10] Shortly thereafter Jarvis began a long correspondence with De Bow about the nature and purpose of the census that was destined to have a major impact upon its quality and utility.

After receiving the statistics that he sought and a friendly reply, Jarvis sent De Bow a twenty-page analysis of existing procedures and suggestions for improvements. Jarvis was specifically concerned with two issues. First, if, as he believed, science was taxonomy, then far greater attention would have to be given to improving census schedules. Consequently, he urged more precise age categories; he insisted that the distinction between pure blacks and mulattoes be extended throughout the census in order to determine whether the latter were more susceptible to disease than either the former or whites; and he suggested a simple but admittedly imperfect procedure to compute average age.

Even more distressing were the medical statistics, for an inappropriate nosology rendered them virtually useless. Referring to the nosologies prepared by both the American Medical Association and William Farr in England, Jarvis called for the adoption of some uniform and scientific system. He also proposed that the data be aggregated in several ways in order to enhance the possibilities of relating a variety of factors. If health was a function of environment and race, for example, then life expectancy tables should be given by region and race as well as by nation. Secondly, Jarvis insisted that the very imperfections of the raw data severely limited the definitive character of the census. The number of deaths reported by the marshalls was far less than the number that had actually occurred, a defect that he attributed to high rates of internal migration. Consequently, Jarvis supported the publication of the mortality tables, but only with an explanatory note "advising the reader not to take it as the whole truth, but to believe these were all the facts that came to the knowledge of the Marshalls."[11]

Jarvis's long communication met with an appreciative response from De Bow, who promptly raised some further methodological problems concerning the best means for estimating the precise number of foreign-born and their descendants in the United States. By this time many native Americans linked social problems and immigration; they saw a causal relationship between the character and culture of immigrants and crime, unemployment, disease, and a deteriorating urban environment. The result was a vigorous effort to gather as much data as possible to illuminate the precise nature of this relationship. Consequently, mid-nineteenth-century censuses, state as well as federal, phrased their questions in terms of native and foreign-born. Conversely, there was no effort to gather data by class and income distribution categories. To put it another way, the census mirrored a prevailing conviction that immigrants (and, to a lesser extent, racial groups) bore a large measure of responsibility for prevailing social ills.

De Bow in his letter expressed concern with Kennedy's estimates of the number of foreign-born and their descendants in the United States. These estimates were based on Jesse Chickering's influential analysis of immigration published in 1848. Chickering's book, ostensibly a study of the extent of immigration, was in reality a warning to his fellow-countrymen. His statistics seemed to lead to the conclusion that within twenty-five years the foreign-born and their descendants would constitute a majority of the population and be capable of controlling the

electoral process. There were, according to Chickering, fundamental differences between natives on the one hand and
foreign-born and their children on the other; the latter defined
liberty as "a licentiousness which has no respect for the rights of
others." Moreover, most foreigners came to America "to benefit themselves, not from any love of us or of our country"; few
of them understood or appreciated their adopted homeland.
The American people, he concluded in somber words, could no
longer avoid giving this subject "their most deliberate
consideration."[12]

In responding to De Bow's concern, Jarvis expressed grave reservations about Kennedy's and Chickering's methodology,
which resulted in an exaggeration of the number of foreign-
born and their descendants in the United States in 1850.[13] The
only way to provide some accurate estimates, wrote Jarvis, was to
determine first the number of incoming immigrants from customs house records and to approximate the remainder. The second step was to estimate the age distribution either from records
or by computation. In the final stage mortality tables could be
applied to determine the probable number of survivors, thus arriving at a realistic estimate for 1850. This method, he pointed
out, gave a smaller total of foreign-born and descendants alive
in 1850 than did the returns of marshalls. The figures of the
marshalls were grossly inaccurate, for language and cultural differences made immigrants reluctant to provide officials with accurate information. Nor were the imperfections in the data
relating to immigrants unique; the number of reported deaths
fell far short of the actual total. In levying this criticism Jarvis
was drawing upon his knowledge of registration statistics, which
enabled him to run a reliability test on the federal census. Imprecision in language also detracted from the usefulness of the
data. The word "adult," to cite one illustration, was nowhere
defined in terms of age; the occupational categories were con-
fusing and led to misleading responses.[14]

At the end of 1853 the seventh census was finally published.
Nearly twelve hundred pages in length, it was a quantitative
and qualitative improvement over its predecessors. Jarvis offered
his congratulations to De Bow, but not without emphasizing
the remaining defects, including the obvious omission of nu-

merous towns and counties. Particularly annoying was the fact that the new census did not correct the glaring errors in the census of 1840. Nevertheless, the improved work augured well for the future.[15]

Early in 1854 Congress ordered De Bow to prepare a new and condensed version of the census. Unhampered by previous commitments, De Bow proceeded to rearrange data in a manner that enhanced its utility. In so doing he continued to call upon Jarvis for advice. The latter responded without hesitation, for he wanted to prevent continued misuse of statistical data. A case in point involved the statistics of pauperism. Although Kennedy had included some material pertaining to this subject in his abstract, the forthcoming compendium seemed to provide an opportunity to shed additional light on the subject, and De Bow began to analyze the returns. Jarvis's interest was aroused when the New York *Herald* used Kennedy's data during the heated congressional debate over slavery in the territories to demonstrate that there was more poverty, insanity, and idiocy in the North than the South. Those Northerners who condemned slavery as a social and moral evil, the *Herald* editorialized, would do well to look at "the white slavery system of the North" first.[16]

Jarvis was angered by the *Herald*'s comments. Aside from his hostility toward slavery, he was incensed at the misrepresentation of the census figures. Kennedy's table, he wrote to De Bow, assumed that pauperism was the same in all the states, whereas in reality it included only those "whom the law compels the public to support." The number of legal paupers, therefore, was merely an expression of state policy; the inclusion of Kennedy's table in the compendium had to be accompanied by a "disclaimer of any inference to be drawn as to the amount of privation without first examining the laws respecting pauperism & the custom of relieving it from the public treasury."[17]

The publication of the compendium in late 1854 was a significant milestone in the evolution of the federal census, for it embodied many of the changes for which Jarvis and others had been fighting. The original census volume provided data by counties and states; the new compendium included the same data reaggregated in far more comprehensive tables as well as additional data from other sources. The thrust of the volume was graphically demonstrated by the large number of comparative and ratio tables. This feature was particularly appealing to those who hoped to convince legislators to follow the lead of statisticians in formulating policy. De Bow's introduction also constituted a firm and articulate defense of a modernized census, for he recommended the establishment of a permanent central statistical office. Although Jarvis's specific contributions to the preparation of the compendium were minimal because his energies during the latter part of the year were devoted to the preparation of the *Report on Insanity,* there is little doubt that his specific criticisms influenced De Bow's discussion of immigrants, black insanity, and pauperism.[18]

III

Given the limitations of size mandated by Congress, De Bow was unable to include in the compendium the statistics of manufactures and mortality. In December 1854, however, the House of Representatives authorized the printing of the mortality statistics in a volume not to exceed three hundred pages. De Bow immediately set to work to prepare a plan for presenting the data.[19]

In a previous communication in August 1853 Jarvis warned of the defects in the census schedules relating to mortality, and shortly thereafter De Bow conceded the validity of these criticisms. Jarvis responded by urging that the table entitled "Number of Deaths" be changed to "Number of Deaths Heard of" in order to convey the impression that the mortality statistics were not thoroughly reliable. In early 1854 Jarvis followed up his previous comments with a longer statement. In examining the proposed form of the mortality statistics, two things had to be kept in mind: how to convey truth, and how to avoid perpetuating error. Regarding the second admonition, it was evident that "no rate of mortality" could even be conjectured from the statistics, nor could any valid comparisons be drawn. To obviate these difficulties it was imperative that a clear statement be included "that *these are only a part of the facts.*" For it was obvious that the published facts would have value only if the reported facts were in the same proportion to the whole. Jarvis then gave a number of suggestions to sharpen the categories used to report the data after this caveat. In closing he offered to prepare a "proper nosological nomenclature" at his home in Dorchester. Given De Bow's recognition that the inadequate appropriation for his department precluded the employment of a medical statistician, it was not surprising that he accepted Jarvis's offer of assistance.[20]

During the spring and summer Jarvis devoted a substantial part of his time to the census. The work proceeded slowly, partly because of the time required in Washington to compile the list of diseases from the returns of the marshalls. By September Jarvis had completed his work and sent a revised nosology based on the one adopted by the American Medical Association in 1847 (in turn based upon Farr's system).[21] Jarvis's nosology was basically derivative in character. His preoccupation with classification was typical of the medical profession both in the United States and abroad. The accumulation of observations about diseases threatened to overwhelm even those on the frontiers of medicine. It was understandable, therefore, that the simplification of accumulated data about disease held considerable appeal. Without the ability to identify similar and dissimilar phenomena there could be no such thing as science. Classification seemed the most appropriate means of bringing order out of chaos. But what system of classification was best? To organize diseases by their causes was impossible; knowledge of specific etiological factors was absent and medical technology had not reached the point where it was possible for physicians to identify diseases by their causes. Hence Jarvis, like his contemporaries, fell back on a nosology based on external symptoms. This created some obvious problems. Fever, for example, was a symptom of innumerable diseases; yet Jarvis listed seven classes of fever (from the general class of fever to specific categories such as intermittent, remittent, ship, scarlet, yellow, and typhoid fever). His faith in the moral and uniform nature of the universe was so firm that he never questioned the basis of his nosological system. His categories were virtually given in nature; all that remained was to discover the relationship between these categories and the external environment. In this respect his concept of research was not fundamentally different from modern social research with its emphasis on classification, collection of data, and application of statistical correlation techniques.

The volume on the mortality statistics that appeared at the end of 1855 incorporated many of Jarvis's proposals, particularly his revision of the nosology of diseases. The limitations of space, however, precluded publication of a table for each state giving the specific disease, age, color, and condition. This omission proved particularly disheartening to Jarvis. Significantly, De Bow's general introduction echoed Jarvis on many points.[22]

Jarvis's reaction to the final product was favorable, for he recognized that the space limitation mandated by Congress prevented the inclusion of more elaborate tables based on further calculations. "Yet it is useless to complain of what we could not have," he wrote to De Bow. "We should rather be thankful for what we have gained."[23] To Jarvis, however, the volume was only a beginning. While the census statistics seemed to provide irrefutable evidence of the nation's growing material and spiritual progress, it was not yet reliable enough for scientists and physicians, and the dangers of misusing possibly invalid data also remained compelling.[24] Conceding that the census of 1850 was a sharp improvement over its six predecessors, Jarvis nevertheless felt that much remained to be done if it were to become the point at which science and policy might be wed in an ideal union.

Publication of the mortality statistics signaled the end of the Seventh Census and the dismantling of the Washington office responsible for the project. But Jarvis's connection with the census of 1850 was not to end for another two decades because of a curious situation that arose in the autumn of 1855. In September of that year Jarvis proposed that he be compensated for the time he had given to the preparation of the census. Between 1853 and 1855 he sent De Bow more than twenty communications totalling over three hundred pages. Jarvis's request came as something of a surprise, if only because no mention of compensation had been made in earlier communications. Nevertheless, De Bow did not think the claim unreasonable. The difficulty was that the appropriation for the census department was exhausted and there were insufficient funds to cover all previous commitments. De Bow suggested that the sum of $1,500 was appropriate, $500 of which represented the labor on the mortality statistics and $1,000 the remainder. He also urged Jarvis to forward a petition to Congress, since there were no funds to pay him.[25]

Jarvis was not completely pleased with De Bow's response, for he thought it inappropriate to file an independent claim for work performed for the government. Given the fact that De Bow was no longer a federal employee, Jarvis had no choice. With De Bow's endorsement and support, he sent his claim to his congressional representative, and also enlisted the aid of Senators Charles Sumner and Henry Wilson. Having decided that he was entitled to compensation, Jarvis was not the type of person who would readily forgo what he felt was due him. But he insisted that his claim be included with others that were outstanding; to do otherwise might weaken his case and convey the implication of special pleading. The case dragged on for several years without any resolution. Just when Congress appeared on the verge of approving the appropriation, the Civil War intervened and the case was postponed indefinitely, much to Jarvis's chagrin.[26]

After the war Jarvis continued to push for congressional action. Having agreed to prepare the volume on the mortality statistics for the census of 1860 (for a stipend), he sought to persuade the secretary of the interior to support his earlier claim. In 1866 Congress once again took up the issue. Much to Jarvis's annoyance, there was opposition to his claim; several representatives thought that a poor precedent would be set because there had been neither an agreement about compensation nor a contract. The bill narrowly passed the House, but the Senate refused to act. Nevertheless, Jarvis refused to become discouraged, and he continued his lobbying efforts. Success finally came in 1874 when Congress passed and the President signed a bill granting him the sum of $1,500.[27]

IV

While fighting to improve the accuracy of the federal census, Jarvis continued his efforts to improve the quality of state and local statistics and even supported the establishment of a Massachusetts census.[28] In 1855 he published a lengthy review of state registration reports analyzing their deficiencies. The Massachusetts reports from 1849 to 1852, he noted, appeared to indicate that urban areas had significantly higher mortality rates than rural areas. But the absence of the age distribution of their respective populations negated any such conclusion. Cities often had younger populations and a higher proportion of children and infants—two groups with extraordinarily high death rates. Life expectancy of specific age groups in urban and rural areas, therefore, might not be affected by differential gross mortality rates. Nor was Jarvis satisfied with tables relating occupation and longevity, especially since no account was taken of broad environmental conditions not specifically related to a particular job. Even more significant was the very imprecision of the occupational categories themselves. "The proper classification," he suggested in tentative terms, "is not according to names, but according to sanitary influence."[29]

Jarvis also attempted to rally organizational support on behalf of the cause of vital statistics. In 1858 he prepared a report for the American Medical Association's Committee on Registration urging member physicians to throw their weight behind improved procedures. Jarvis was also active within the American Statistical Association and the Massachusetts Medical Society, and pushed both organizations to throw their weight behind the effort to improve the state registration system, then the most advanced in the nation.[30]

If he was distressed by the inadequacies of registration procedures, he was angered by individuals who utilized inaccurate statistics to draw definitive conclusions. Jarvis was cognizant of the varied uses to which data could be put. Viewed in the abstract, knowledge was neutral and objective. In practice, however, knowledge had operational consequences. Conscious and unconscious prejudices, when combined with inaccurate or incomplete data, could have detrimental results for individuals

and society as a whole. It was therefore imperative that taxonomical and data imperfections be exposed. The rapid human
and economic growth of American society rendered even more
pressing the necessity for objective knowledge and dispassionate
analysis in order to formulate appropriate policies. Curiously
enough, Jarvis never envisaged that his analysis could be turned
around and used to undermine his own nosology.

In 1859 Jarvis once again used the pages of the *American
Journal of the Medical Sciences* to express his feelings when he
reviewed James Wynne's *Report on the Vital Statistics of the
United States.* A Baltimore physician, Wynne prepared his
study at the request of the Mutual Life Insurance Company of
New York. Since 1854 the company had divided the United
States into geographical sections and established differential
premium rates. Southerners paid higher rates, which led to frequent charges of discrimination. Wynne's report, written by a
border state physician, seemed to vindicate the company's insis-
tence that differential mortality rates were responsible for the
existing rate structure.[31]

Jarvis's private comments were unfavorable. Wynne, he told
the editor, made use of only a limited range of "authorities &
facts." He had not examined the English registration reports
and was obliged to accept some authorities at second hand.
Overall the book added "less than it should, to statistical science, & fails to establish its principles on a surer foundation."
The work also contained errors, the most important being the
inference from a previously published study of English Friendly
Societies "that the poor do not suffer from their condition, circumstances, & habits."[32] In his published version Jarvis was
somewhat gentler. Indeed, much of the article was devoted to a
review of his earlier analyses of the validity of registration and
census statistics.[33]

The collection of data, however important, was only a means
to an end; Jarvis did not lose sight of the larger goal of shaping
policy through the application of scientific knowledge. His interest in the census and registration, therefore, was rarely divorced from his concern with social problems and social policy.
A specific case in point involved the indiscriminate manner in
which society imprisoned convicted lawbreakers. Crime, noted

Jarvis, had "manifold and protean forms," and its origins were "equally varied." Yet society assumed that criminal acts had an identical source. Consequently, imprisonment was the universal and characteristic mode of punishment, the only difference being the duration of incarceration. "The law in selecting the means of punishing crime," he complained, "goes not behind the fact and utterly ignores its inner origin; and justice in determining the measure of the retribution, is equally regardless and unphilosophical. Whether the criminals be male or female, malignant or wanton, selfish or self sacrificing, they are all condemned to the same punishment, varied only in quantity."[34]

The inferior quality of data found in prison reports, Jarvis argued, was partly responsible for the inadequate public policies dealing with crime. Sex, age, nativity, types of crime, and prior personal histories were all important variables in understanding and changing criminal behavior; the absence of such knowledge obviously hampered policy analysis and formulation. Did unrestricted immigration bring criminal types to the United States, thereby causing a sharp increase in the crime rate that exceeded the growth of population? Or was the involvement of immigrants in illegal activities a result of living in a strange new environment? Only a careful analysis of the "conditions and circumstances of the offences and . . . criminal acts and the connection of these together" would illuminate the causes of crime and the "effects of remedial measures."[35]

To prove his point Jarvis examined tens of thousands of male and female crimes. Males were invariably committed to prison for crimes against persons and property. Such acts involved the use of intellect in the sense that the criminal was the beneficiary and the victim the injured party. Females were committed for intemperance, lasciviousness, and prostitution. Such crimes grew out of the indulgence of bodily appetites and passions and injured only the guilty party. Although both sexes were treated in the same manner, the results were quite different. Imprisonment for a male thief served a useful function; it demonstrated that the act was a costly one, and that honesty was the path to be followed. Incarceration for acts involving the passions and appetites, however, served no purpose; it merely resulted in a much higher recidivist rate for women (as compared with men). "Is it not then both unphilosophical and unnatural," asked Jarvis, "to treat these moral disorders, so diverse in their origin, & in their relation to the human constitution, with the same remedy with the hope of healing them?" Accurate crime statistics, he concluded, could aid in distinguishing special cases from general principles, thereby providing the basis for sound and effective policies.[36]

Fascination with aggregate data reinforced Jarvis's desire to take an active role in public affairs, particularly when his knowledge could influence the outcome. In 1855, for example, he acceded to a request from the Dorchester Board of Health and prepared a code of health laws that was promptly adopted. Interestingly enough, Jarvis gave the board wide latitude and authority over all matters that affected public health. Under his code the board had broad powers of inspection; it could compel the removal of nuisances, ban the possession or sale of unwholesome or contaminated food, require suitable privies for all inhabitants and dwellings, maintain minimum housing standards, and regulate all unhealthful and offensive occupations as well as cemeteries and burial grounds. A few years later Jarvis was called upon to provide statistical confirmation for a memorial to the state legislature opposing the filling in and later use of the Back Bay area in Boston.[37]

Although eager to provide aid for a variety of projects, Jarvis grew increasingly dissatisfied with the policy-making process. Too many important decisions had been made on the basis of ignorance, prejudice, or simple common sense, none of which gave rise to policies that achieved the desired results. His role in helping to revamp the census of 1850 only reinforced his determination to find more effective means of convincing Americans that they had everything to gain and little to lose by making policy on the basis of objective and impartial facts.

7

Public Policy, Medicine, and Government

By the end of the 1850s Jarvis could look back at his achievements with pride and satisfaction. The inner doubts that
had plagued him in the years following his graduation from
medical school were now but a distant and shadowy memory.
His work as a psychiatrist, statistician, and social analyst had
given him a national reputation. Indeed, the success that he
achieved in overcoming early adversity strengthened his faith in
the possibilities of continued progress. No evil was so extreme as
to be ineradicable; no person was so sinful as to be unredeem-
able; no illness was so inevitable as to be unpreventable; no
situation was so far gone as to be beyond control. A dispassionate analysis of social problems within a divinely ordained moral
system provided humanity with the tools, knowledge, and wisdom to create a better world.

During the 1860s, therefore, Jarvis's confidence in the future
helped to sustain his involvement with social and medical problems. In his eyes the orderly nature of the physical world was a
reality; he never considered the possibility that the human mind
might merely impose coherence upon the disorderly facts of
nature. His views led him to codify in precise terms the respective
roles of government on the one hand and medicine and science
on the other. Social and class conflict, he implied, was abnormal
and occurred only when human beings were uninformed or mis-
informed. When men possessed knowledge and wisdom, proper
policies would become self-evident because of their given quality. The function of medicine was simply to discover a preexist-

ing order. Similarly, the role of government was not to mediate between competing groups or to impose controls, but rather to disseminate eternal truths among a rational citizenry. And reality was best expressed in statistical terms, for statistics was the language of a divine power. In describing reality, science and medicine simultaneously defined the policies that ought to govern any society. Progress would follow if government confined its activities to the discovery of truth and education of its citizens.

Jarvis's varied activities reflected the faith that had sustained him since youth. In 1860 he satisfied a lifelong desire to travel abroad and to meet co-workers from other countries who shared similar views. Not even the Civil War could dispel his faith in the possibilities of further progress; the conflict provided an opportunity to apply sanitarian principles and thereby reduce morbidity and mortality rates among the armed forces. Nor did the war in any way dampen his concern with vital statistics or mental illness. Within his native state he led abortive efforts to induce the legislature to establish a state board of health and to alter public policy as it related to the mentally ill.

Paradoxically, Jarvis's influence over events declined rather than increased during the 1860s. His involvement in public affairs was predicated upon the assumption that truth and conflict were incompatible, and that appropriate policies were inherent in the natural order, waiting only to be discovered. Few of his countrymen, however, shared such views. In the America of the 1860s conflict was the norm rather than the exception; few groups hesitated to use government to promote their own interests, and still fewer were willing to abrogate to intellectuals or scientists the right to make authoritative decisions. In a pluralistic society where the mechanisms of government were diffuse and authority fragmented, success came to those who were willing to take part in the give and take of political compromise and forge alliances based on mutual self-interest rather than eternal principle.

Yet Jarvis remained oblivious to the dilemmas that grew out of his philosophy of government. He never recognized that others might hold a vision of the good society quite different from his own. Like many intellectuals, he believed that the categories of good and evil were clear and unequivocal; once discovered they could not be transformed by human volition. This belief hampered his efforts to modify public policy, for the very traits that were conducive to his statistical research often proved a liability in the political arena. Consequently, Jarvis achieved his greatest success and influence as a publicist for statistics and preventive medicine; as a molder of policy he was less successful.

I

The outward success that Jarvis achieved by the mid-1850s was accompanied by an inner contentment. His orderly life in Dorchester created an environment conducive to professional activities. Perhaps his only disappointment was his continued inability to secure a hospital superintendency, a position that eluded his grasp for over two decades. In 1856 and 1857 he was considered for two such offices but failed to receive an offer. When the legislature seemed on the verge of establishing a permanent board of state charities in 1859, Luther V. Bell immediately wrote to Jarvis to ascertain his interest in being considered for the position of executive officer. Jarvis responded affirmatively. Aside from personal ambition, he wanted to relieve his wife of the often onerous burden of caring for mentally ill patients in their home. The failure of the legislature to act laid this matter to rest.[1]

Years of work had brought Jarvis into contact with like-minded figures in England and on the continent. Yet he had never traveled beyond the continental boundaries of the United States (with the exception of a brief Canadian sojourn) and observed conditions elsewhere. Early in 1860, however, a fortuitous event provided an unparalleled opportunity to fulfil a long-standing ambition and at the same time not to incur personal expense or loss of income. Toward the end of February the wife of a wealthy merchant proposed that Jarvis accompany them on a trip abroad. Her husband was suffering from some mental problems, and she decided (probably after consulting with Dr. Jacob Bigelow) that an extended foreign trip was in order. Jarvis immediately accepted the offer. In return for his medical services, he would receive a stipend of $1,200 per quarter and all of his expenses would be paid by the family.[2] The fact that the fourth International Statistical Congress was scheduled to meet in London in July made the trip even more desirable.

On March 7 Jarvis sailed from Boston. After a tedious trip of nearly thirteen days, the ship landed in Liverpool. For Jarvis the experience of setting foot on English soil was exhilirating, although home, as he wrote to Almira, "is never far from my thoughts." The day after his arrival he visited the Rainhill lunatic hospital, which was located about nine miles outside the city. Jarvis was most impressed by the relative absence of physical and mechanical restraint; violent patients were either put under the care of an extra attendant or else sent to their rooms. Irish patients, Jarvis observed, presented some of the very same problems that they did in the United States; they were "the most difficult to manage, the least curable & most prone to sink into dementia." In walking through the streets of Liverpool he was struck by the relative coarseness of women and the lack of vigor manifested by the poor and destitute.[3]

From Liverpool the group proceeded to Chester. Medieval structures, especially churches, caught Jarvis's imagination, for they portrayed a society long since gone. Most interesting were his conversations with educated Englishmen, one of whom described the large Irish population in unflattering terms. Jarvis, however, thought that only the "best" of the Irish migrated to America, where they were "led to do better than they would here or at [their] home." From Chester the party went to Malvern, located about nine miles from Worcester. Jarvis visited overnight at the Worcestershire lunatic asylum, where the superintendent gave him a gracious and kind welcome. Jarvis was especially impressed with the degree and manner in which patients were kept occupied. "I thought then of the halls at our Worcester [hospital], so full, through the day, of the listless, lifeless, thoughtless, deathly patients, whose torpid bodies & torpid minds seemed to be daily gathering more torpor, because no one, no officer, or attendant, no system, no efficient hope had drawn them out to work, to dance, to sing, to do anything sanely." American mental hospitals, in his opinion, compared unfavorably with their English counterparts.[4]

Toward the end of May Jarvis fulfilled a long-standing ambition when he visited London. There he received a friendly greeting from figures with whom he had corresponded for many years, including Dr. Forbes Winslow, the members of the London Statistical Society, and the Commissioners in Lunacy. The highlight of this brief visit was an overnight stay with the distinguished John Conolly, head of the Hanwell asylum and the leading exponent of the nonrestraint system in the care and treatment of the insane.[5]

In June, Jarvis visited Birmingham and Oxford and paid a return trip to London, where the Statistical Society arranged a dinner for him at which William Farr was present. On June 23 Jarvis's entire party moved to London, where he took every opportunity to visit welfare, penal, and medical institutions. His most depressing moment came when he wandered through St. Giles, where the populace lived in poverty and misery. "Everything," he wrote to his wife, "indicated a lower life, a life steeped in poverty, in error, in degradation. . . . Here were the gatherings of sin and destitution and self-indulgence. Here low appetite revelled and passion ruled. Here moral sentiment found no quickening of life. Here children were born in filth, raised in sin and lived in corruption."[6]

Such depressing observations, however, were rare, for his reception as a leading physician and statistician was exhilarating. Equally satisfying was his sense of triumph as an American. Although never demonstrating overt hostility toward English and European colleagues, Jarvis may have harbored unconscious feelings of antipathy that grew out of his perception that American medicine and science lagged behind. Acceptance as an American, therefore, may have helped to assuage any sense of inferiority about his country. At a dinner of the Law Amendment Society, Lord Brougham, whose own catholic interests in innumerable causes spanned more than half a century, toasted Jarvis and asked him to say a few words. The event seemed symbolic. "*I* speak to the English chancellors, lords, judges, parliamentary members, lawyers, men of note and high renown and cultivation!" Jarvis exulted in a letter to Almira. "I, the Dorchester doctor, speak to that audience! Yet there I was in the presence of these men and called upon; so I rose and they sa-

luted me cordially." At this very moment Jarvis chose to extol
the greatness of his native land and to attribute American power
and greatness to the universal intelligence so assiduously cultivated among its citizens.[7] Private meetings with others, including Edwin Chadwick and Florence Nightingale, only reinforced
his growing confidence in himself and his country.[8]

The high point of the trip came in mid-July, when the fourth
International Statistical Congress brought together distinguished
statisticians and social researchers from more than a dozen coun-
tries. The only official American delegate was Augustus Baldwin
Longstreet, the well-known author of *Georgia Scenes* (1835),
jurist, and college president; Jarvis represented the American
Statistical Association (although in London he convinced
George M. Dallas, the American minister to England, and
Longstreet, to accredit him as a national delegate).[9]

When the congress opened on July 16 Jarvis became embroiled in a bitter controversy. In his opening remarks Lord
Brougham called attention to the fact that Martin R. Delany, a
black, was present. An early exponent of black nationalism, a
champion of black people, and a physician whose attendance at
the Harvard Medical School caused a major conflict within that
institution, Delany received a royal appointment as a delegate
to the congress. Brougham's remarks were answered by Delany,
who expressed his appreciation and then concluded that he was
merely "a man." Longstreet immediately withdrew from the
meeting, claiming that Brougham had insulted the American
people. Dallas, who was present at the session, supported Longstreet, and the incident immediately blossomed into a major
diplomatic controversy involving both governments.[10]

As an American representative, Jarvis was unable to remain
aloof. A long-standing opponent of slavery, he nevertheless subordinated his own inclinations and attempted to play the role of
mediator, for he did not want a divisive issue to detract from the
work of the congress. Brougham informed Jarvis that he had not
intended to reproach his American brethren; he had simply
pointed to Delany as an example of how far a member of a race
hitherto regarded as inferior, ignorant, and uncivilized might
advance. Although Brougham repeated these words in public,

Longstreet and Dallas held fast to their position; Jarvis was unable to induce them to alter their stand.[11]

During the week-long meeting Jarvis took an active part both in the discussions and formal presentations. In his initial talk he described the state of statistical research in America and his own work. He followed this presentation with papers that summarized statistics dealing with the relationship between occupation and longevity and also repeated his earlier findings on the comparative liability of males and females to various types of crime. In his concluding paper he appealed for an international effort to collect vital statistics in order to shed light on the factors that contributed to human deficiencies. During the deliberations Jarvis also prevailed on the delegates to adopt a resolution urging all hospitals for the insane to adopt a common classification system in order to collect comparable data that would clarify etiology and the effectiveness of various therapies.[12]

The work of the congress, pleasurable in itself, was relieved by several rewarding social engagements that bolstered Jarvis's outlook. "This week, Almira," he wrote in glowing terms, "has been one of the pleasantest of my life. Here I was among the men of all the earth whose minds and tastes and pursuits are most similar to my own; and to be thrown into such familiar association with them, to be received so cordially and readily, to find myself so well known and to float along so easily with them, is certainly a blessing very pleasant to my heart and may I ever be thankful for it."[13]

Following the close of the congress, Jarvis proceeded to Dover and then to France for a hurried visit. He found Paris a "city of beauty, grace, magnificence, voluptuousness and vanity!" While there he visited the Salpêtrière, perhaps the largest hospital in the world, and then spent some time with Jean C.M.F.J. Boudin, whose work on the geographical distribution of disease several years earlier perpetuated the errors of the census of 1840. The trip to France proved all too brief, and after a few days on the continent Jarvis returned to London on July 27. Four days later he arrived in Edinburgh, where he received a warm welcome from Dr. Thomas Laycock, whose recent two-volume work *Mind and Brain* anticipated the study of unconscious cerebration, and Sir James Coxe, a member of the Board of Lunacy for Scotland. Both men guided him on a tour of Scottish mental hospitals. On August 4 Jarvis embarked on a ship leaving Liverpool for the United States, and twelve days later he landed in New York.[14]

Aside from obvious personal satisfactions, Jarvis's trip proved significant in other ways. His ties to colleagues in other countries were cemented by personal contacts. His visits to more than a dozen mental hospitals in England, Scotland, and France enabled him to observe firsthand the British system of nonrestraint; in the years to come he would take part in the developing controversy over its applicability in American hospitals. To be sure, not all of his observations were uncritical. He preferred the more fluid social structure of the United States to the fixed and hierarchical organization of English society. English landowning and tenancy practices encouraged a paternal relationship between lower and upper classes that clearly favored the latter.[15] Such reservations, however, in no way detracted from Jarvis's enthusiasm, nor did his commitment to his native land inhibit a receptivity to learn and to profit from the experiences of others. Within his perceptual framework nationalism was a beneficent force compatible with human progress. A consistent adherence to a broad environmentalism prevented him from joining other Bay State natives who were becoming increasingly pessimistic about the future and who would ultimately create a racial ideology based on fear of the future.[16]

II

Stimulated by contacts with statisticians and sanitarians at the congress, Jarvis returned home eager to continue his efforts to improve governmental data gathering activities. A few months later an opportunity presented itself when the Boston Sanitary Association, with the support of both the American Statistical Association and the Massachusetts Medical Society, voted to petition the Massachusetts legislature to establish a state board of health. Founded a year or two earlier, the Boston Sanitary Association brought together prominent Bostonians for discussions of contemporary problems. Its first public meeting was not held until January 1861, at which time Jarvis gave an address that called attention to the social and economic inequities of urban life that promoted high morbidity and mortality rates among the lower classes while permitting the rich to escape unscathed "by virtue of cleanliness, exercise, wholesome food, and other advantages derived from their position." Shortly thereafter Jarvis prepared the memorial, which was signed by Josiah Quincy, Jr., and Dr. Josiah Curtis and presented to the legislature in mid-February.[17] Nearly a decade had passed since Shattuck first proposed such a board. During the intervening years there was little or no interest in the project. The absence of virulent epidemics and preoccupation with the developing sectional conflict overshadowed concern with disease and death. Indeed, the four National Quarantine and Sanitary Conventions held between 1857 and 1860 (the last in Boston) reflected a mood of optimism; most of the delegates were convinced that environmental measures could eliminate many of the major scourges still afflicting humanity. The redoubtable Dr. Jacob Bigelow, still active in his mid-seventies, declared that Americans were standing on the threshold of a new era; he looked forward to a time when sanitary science would all but replace clinical medicine.[18]

Written by Jarvis, the memorial of the Boston Sanitary Association echoed Bigelow's optimistic affirmation. Jarvis called for no striking expansion of governmental authority over the lives of citizens; in this respect he rejected the allegation that the maintenance of social order and prosperity was dependent upon the supervision of the American people by a beneficent and enlightened elite. The role of government, he insisted, was to promote health, an objective that could be attained by careful statistical analysis of morbidity and mortality patterns and a broad program of education that appealed to the self-interest of people. A board of health would employ rational persuasion, not compulsion. It would have three basic functions: to superintend the registration of births, marriages, and deaths; to conduct the decennial census; and to assume visitorial and supervisory authority over state hospitals and welfare institutions, particularly in regard to the reporting of statistical data.[19]

The proposal could hardly have come at a less propitious moment; the clouds of civil war were already visible on the horizon. Jarvis attempted to persuade Governor John A. Andrew to support the legislation, and Josiah Curtis, fearful that lethargy plus active opposition would result in the bill's defeat, suggested an intensive lobbying campaign. Curtis was not sanguine about the eventual outcome; the lateness of the session, the prevalence of "cliques," and "corruption" all posed formidable threats. Curtis's fears (if not his reasons) were justified. Despite a favorable report by a joint special committee, the legislature took no action. During the succeeding two years other efforts to establish a state board of health proved equally futile.[20]

The failure of the legislature to act did not in any way imply a denial of the principles of state responsibility for health-related matters; laws dealing with contaminated and adulterated food and the regulation of the noxious trades were routinely enacted during the 1860s. The lukewarm reception accorded Jarvis's pet scheme was due rather to other factors. Outside of Boston there seemed little enthusiasm for the project. "The great trouble," observed a Lancaster resident in a letter to Jarvis, "is that country members [of the legislature] look upon the whole thing as a Boston concern and not understanding its importance, are disposed to give it the go by." Even Josiah Bartlett admitted that he did not understand why such a board was necessary; municipal officials acting as such a board invariably performed effectively. Jarvis himself believed that the most potent opposition came from the secretary of state's office, which feared a loss of jobs if registration was transferred to the jurisdiction of another agency.[21]

Perhaps the fatal impediment to passage of the bill was its implied rationale. Jarvis argued that in the long run the state would benefit from the knowledge that would accrue from quantified data. Yet he was unable to demonstrate any specific relationship between an effective system of registration on the one hand and the prevention of disease on the other. Legislators, who by this time were preoccupied with the social and economic costs of dependency, disease, and crime, could see few direct linkages in Jarvis's plan and therefore were not disposed to authorize expenditures for a new state board of health. Although the Massachusetts Medical Society endorsed the proposal, the mass of practicing physicians in the state ignored the project; their energies were absorbed in caring for their patients, and they showed little concern for preventing diseases whose nature and etiology had yet to be established.[22] Interestingly enough, in 1863 the legislature established a board of state charities, partly because of a generalized fear that immigrants were threatening the homogeneity and well-being of society and partly in the hope of reducing welfare costs. Whereas the legislature's action reflected pessimism and fear, Jarvis's proposal was based on an entirely different assumption, namely, that enlightened self-interest could contribute toward the creation of a healthy and just society.[23] Perhaps for this reason the governor responded negatively when Jarvis's name was proposed by Howe for membership on the new board of state charities.[24]

III

When the Civil War commenced in the spring of 1861, neither Northern nor Southern authorities had given any thought to the organization of medical services in their armed forces. But the extraordinarily large number of troops on both sides created serious problems involving the treatment of battle-related injuries as well as the maintenance of sanitary standards in military camps. The huge number of deaths from wounds and disease led physicians and sanitary reformers to offer their services to the government in order to reduce a mortality rate that threatened to destroy the effectiveness of the military. The result was a debate among sanitarians over the precise measures that were required—a debate that ultimately involved large constitutional issues concerning the degree to which public power could be used to foster and to protect public interests.[25]

When fighting began Jarvis was too old to enter the Union Army. In addition, he was not fond of surgery (the most vital specialty of military medicine), and long before had rejected most prevailing therapies. Therapeutic skepticism, however, was not synonymous with a laissez faire fatalism. On the contrary, Jarvis was convinced that decisive government action could sharply reduce morbidity and mortality among soldiers. Three months after the commencement of hostilities he joined with Howe and C.C. Felton in presenting a petition to Congress urging the establishment of a board of military health and the official recognition of the United States Sanitary Commission.[26]

Written by Jarvis, the petition noted that the greatest danger to soldiers came not from actual warfare, but from "personal condition and habits." Humanitarian considerations aside, military effectiveness alone required the diligent application of sanitary principles. To this end the petitioners urged the federal government to establish a permanent board of health to inspect the living conditions of troops and to offer advice to military commanders. The petition also urged Congress to recognize the sanitary commission, and grant it powers of inspection, funds, and partial autonomy.[27]

Unlike other sanitarians who were demanding greater statutory authority in order to replace a vague humanitarianism with an organized and efficient system, Jarvis maintained his long-held conviction that rational men, when presented with valid principles and knowledge, would recognize their true interests and act accordingly. Consequently, he did not propose the creation of formal bureaucratic structures with specific enforcement powers. In this respect he remained closer to the tradition of voluntarism than to the newer belief that philanthropy had to rest on a "scientific" and organizational foundation.

Despite widespread concern with the health of the armed forces, Congress took no action on the petition. Although the war was only three months old, the army and sanitary commission were already engaged in heated and acrimonious conflict. Neither was particularly enthusiastic at the prospect of still another rival. Nor did Jarvis or his colleagues possess the organizational abilities and support necessary for favorable congressional action. The sanitary commission, moreover, was a predominantly New York operation, and there was no evidence that its leaders were willing to share their prerogatives. Finally, Jarvis's proposal probably had little appeal for figures like Henry W. Bellows and Frederick Law Olmsted who were committed to structural rather than voluntaristic solutions.

Although disappointed by congressional inaction, Jarvis did not abandon his interest in reducing military mortality rates.

Toward the end of 1862 he published a lengthy article in the prestigious *Atlantic Monthly* on the "Sanitary Condition of the Army" that condemned in strong language the refusal of military authorities to observe proper sanitary and environmental safeguards. Morbidity and mortality rates were far higher among soldiers than civilians. Nations, he observed more in sorrow than anger, were prepared to inflict death and injury on their opponents, "but they seem neither to look nor to prepare for sickness and death in their camps." Citing the results of the British reorganization of its army following the Crimean War, Jarvis urged that more diligent application of sanitary principles could enhance the effectiveness of the army and reduce the dangers of sickness and death to comparable civilian levels.[28]

So thorough was Jarvis's presentation that Isaac Ray immediately sent an enthusiastic letter of congratulations. "I hope you will not stop here," Ray added. "There are other cognate subjects on which the light of a sound philosophy and of full & accurate statistics, is almost equally necessary, & I know of nobody more competent to furnish that light than you."[29] The appearance of the article was the occasion of an invitation by Governor John A. Andrew asking Jarvis to visit military installations in the Bay State and report on their sanitary condition. During October and November and again in March Jarvis traveled throughout Massachusetts inspecting facilities. His public assessments were enthusiastic and optimistic; his private ones were less sanguine. Unlike other sanitarians, Jarvis was reluctant to commit himself to institutional solutions imposed by men whose authority was derived from the possession of technical knowledge and skills; he remained committed to a voluntaristic ideology. On the other hand, he was cognizant of the difficulties of convincing people to act in ways commensurate with self-interest. The position of sanitary inspector, he complained privately, was "an irresponsible and a gratuitous office. I had no authority to direct, nor power to alter if improvement seemed necessary." Others would resolve the dilemma by opting for greater professional authority and autonomy, but Jarvis remained wedded to his faith in human rationality.[30]

Jarvis's article must have made a favorable impression upon the sanitary commission; it asked him to fill one of their inspectorships of hospitals in the fall of 1862. In spite of organizational conflict between the commission and the Army's medical bureau, Jarvis accepted the invitation without hesitation.[31] The illness of his wife and the presence of several insane patients in his home prevented him from assuming his new position for nearly six months. By April 9, 1863, however, Almira's health had improved, and Jarvis left on a trip that kept him away from home for a month. During his journey he inspected thirty-nine hospitals in the Midwest and seven more in Washington, Philadelphia, and New York. Upon completion of the tour he submitted a report of about 250 pages summarizing his findings. The journey proved a financial loss, for expenses exceeded compensation. More troubling was the fact that the report had no visible impact. Jarvis had assumed that Dr. Henry G. Clark (a fellow Bostonian who acted as inspector-in-chief) would forward his written report to Elisha Harris in New York, but this was apparently not done. Nor was Jarvis's experience unique; Edwin M. Snow encountered a similar situation. In actuality Clark prepared a general summary of the findings of the inspectors, but bureaucratic complexities hid this fact from sight.[32]

IV

While active in a variety of activities, Jarvis never lost his concern for the social and medical problems of mental illness. He continued to be active in the Association of Medical Superintendents. Although some of his colleagues were seeking to define in a precise manner the essential attributes of a professional identity, Jarvis continued to see the role of psychiatry in educational terms. Nor was he willing to create organizational barriers that might impede the broad-based coalition that he felt was so necessary for the promotion of the general welfare. Still seeking utilitarian generalizations about the etiology of insanity, he was instrumental in establishing a system that guaranteed a more comprehensive distribution of the annual reports of mental hospitals, thereby making possible the cumulation and comparison of experiences.[33]

Interest in national issues in no way inhibited concern with state and local concerns. When the general court in 1858 moved to codify all of the acts and resolves enacted during the previous two decades, Jarvis immediately entered the picture. While preparing the *Report on Insanity* he became convinced that existing legal procedures for commitment of patients were inadequate. After reading the proposed codification, he began to sketch out a series of modifications that he presented in a long article in the *Monthly Law Reporter* in 1859.

What astounded Jarvis were the inconsistencies that the new code perpetuated. Its provisions stipulated four methods of commitment to public hospital. The courts were empowered to commit any "furiously mad" person whose behavior threatened public peace and safety. Three other groups—justices of the peace, overseers of the poor, and hospital trustees—had authority to commit specific categories: nonresident insane, town pauper insane, and recent insane persons, respectively. Yet these four categories comprised perhaps fewer than half the total number of insane persons in the state. The precise language of the law, moreover, implied that an individual not falling within one of these classes could not receive the benefits of hospitalization. Jarvis pointed out that the restrictive nature of the law promoted a peculiar but benevolent collusion between judges and families in order to permit the admission of individuals who did not meet the rigid requirements mandated in existing legislation. While no abuses had been uncovered, it was evident that the legal position of hospital superintendents was potentially precarious, since few patients who had been admitted were actually "furiously mad" or posed a threat to others.

In order to end such collusion and also to make hospital facilities available to all classes, Jarvis proposed wide ranging changes. Conceding that deprivation of personal liberty was "one of the greatest sufferings that can be inflicted on man, and among the greatest infringements of his rights," he nevertheless rejected the claim that involuntary confinement violated basic human rights. The exercise of such rights, he implied, was dependent upon a degree of rationality that by definition was absent in many cases of mental disease. Examinations leading to commitment, therefore, involved neither legal nor judicial questions "but a pathological question that is to be answered in the case of insanity . . . by the physicians alone, by men who have been educated and trained to investigate and discern the various phases and manifestations of human health." Endorsing a proposal made by Isaac Ray nearly a decade earlier, Jarvis urged the legislature to establish regional commissions (each including a physician and a magistrate) with the power to decide questions of sanity and with statutory commitment authority. Finally, he urged that county facilities for the harmless insane (whose existence was authorized in 1836 and 1842) be abolished.[34] Jarvis's plea for revision of the laws pertaining to insanity, however, went unheeded, and the general court enacted a new code in 1860 in the form proposed by the commissioners.[35]

Shortly thereafter Jarvis's efforts on behalf of legal reform received support from an unexpected quarter. By this time mental hospitals had come under fire from critics who believed that commitment laws failed to safeguard the rights of patients. In 1862 Samuel E. Sewall, a prominent figure and a trustee of the Worcester hospital, petitioned the legislature in the hope of stimulating passage of a law that would protect the insane against arbitrary action. Sewall received the implicit support of Governor Andrew, who characterized existing laws in his annual address as "defective by reason of incompleteness, inconsistencies, and contradictions." The issue was referred to a special legislative committee.[36]

The testimony before the committee revealed differences between those who were concerned with the legal rights of patients and those who feared that new legislation might diminish chances for admission and limit the ability of hospital superintendents to provide appropriate therapeutic and custodial care. During the committee's deliberations Jarvis was called upon to testify and to prepare a new draft law governing admission procedures and internal administration of public hospitals. After considerable debate the general court enacted a new law in the spring of 1862 that embodied many of the suggestions first proposed by Jarvis in 1859. Specifically, the statute dropped the earlier section that gave to the courts the authority to commit persons "furiously mad" who threatened public safety. In its place the legislature substituted a section that gave judges the right to commit to any state hospital "any insane person who, in their opinion, is a proper subject for its treatment or custody.'' But in all such cases the evidence and certificate of ''at least two respectable physicians'' was required ''to establish the fact of insanity.'' The law implicitly rejected the allegation that insane persons were being deprived of their basic civil rights by the arbitrary action of others. Jarvis was pleased with the final result, particularly because the legislature had interposed no barrier that might have diminished the authority of hospital superintendents. The most effective safeguard for the patient's welfare lay in the character of the superintendent; he had few doubts that incompetency could remain long undetected. The net effect of the new law, aside from establishing certain procedural safeguards, was to diminish collusion between courts and families, and to make the facilities of public hospitals available to all classes.[37]

The new law, however, did not satisfy some critics. At the beginning of 1863 Sewall and twenty others again presented a petition demanding changes in commitment procedures in order to prevent the law from becoming ''the instruments of oppression.'' The result was the creation of a new three-member commission to examine the laws relating to insanity. During their deliberations the members called upon Jarvis and Ray for aid and advice. In their report the commissioners urged the state to adopt a series of procedural safeguards (including the establishment of a commission with powers to rectify unjustified commitments and to discharge patients). Jarvis's influence upon the commission was evident on every page, for it rejected all calls to regulate the internal management of mental hospitals and sharply criticized certain features of state policy that favored the immigrant insane and discriminated against the native insane. The report led to the adoption of a new statute in 1864 that provided additional safeguards to prevent illegal detention in public hospitals and laid down certain regulations for private institutions.[38]

Jarvis's interest in public policy was not confined simply to modes of commitment. On the contrary, his concern with this problem had arisen from his conviction that many individuals who could have benefitted from institutional care and treatment were excluded because of the practical operations of the law. Be-

ginning with his appointment by Governor Andrew as a trustee
of the Worcester State Lunatic Hospital in 1861, he launched a
campaign to transform the manner in which the state financed
institutional care of the insane. His initial appointment was undoubtedly in recognition of his long services to the commonwealth. Certainly the governor never anticipated that Jarvis
would use his position as a vehicle for change. In this respect
Andrew was in error, for Jarvis interpreted the function of the
board of trustees in its original and literal sense, namely, as the
governing body that set policy. Such a vision was quite at variance with the actual role of trustees, most of whom acquiesced in
the transfer of effective authority to the superintendent and saw
their own role in honorific terms.[39]

Jarvis's letter of acceptance anticipated an active role. Thank-
ing Andrew for the appointment, he asked for a meeting to
discuss "the very remarkable way, in which our Lunatic Hospitals are given first to the Irish insane, & to the question of the
propriety or generosity in compelling our own disordered brethren and sisters to associate in the wards of these institutions,
with these foreigners & with criminals from whom they would
shrink, if in health, if they could help themselves." In raising
these issues Jarvis was reflecting the growing concern with the
seemingly endless proliferation of public welfare institutions
and the ensuing increases in expenditures. To some observers
the disproportionately high percentage of foreign-born paupers
in state mental hospitals threatened the health, tranquility, and
well-being of the commonwealth. Fear of immigrants was mirrored in the activities of the board of alien commissioners, an
agency established by the legislature in 1851 for the expressed
purpose of dealing with dependent immigrants.[40]

From the outset it was clear that Jarvis would play an atypical
role. Few of the trustees devoted much time to the hospital's affairs, preferring instead to leave them in the hands of the superintendent. The monthly meetings of the board were as much
social as they were business gatherings. Unlike fellow trustees,
Jarvis paid regular visits to the hospital and spent time with patients, sometimes remaining overnight. He insisted on being
kept informed about finances and the composition of the patient population. No detail was too small to be overlooked.

When the superintendent was elected a Worcester alderman, Jarvis immediately questioned the propriety of this action and emphasized that the board specifically defined the position of superintendent as a full-time job.[41]

In the autumn of 1862 Jarvis was assigned the task of preparing the annual report of the trustees. In the past such statements were largely pro forma and brief in length (sometimes three pages). Jarvis, however, seized the occasion to prepare a document of no less than forty-seven printed pages. In addition to an extended discussion of the nature of insanity, he emphasized an issue that he had raised earlier in the *Report on Insanity*—the manner in which Massachusetts financed institutional care of the insane. Under the law of 1832 the state distinguished between three categories of patients: those who were committed because they represented a danger to the community; those paupers who were not dangerous and who could be committed if their places of residence paid for their support; and those private cases whose families could afford to pay for their upkeep. The law gave the state responsibility for all mentally ill persons not having a legal residence in a particular town. The amount paid by the state was fixed by the legislature. Municipalities were required to pay a sum equal to the cost of supporting their insane paupers, and presumably private patients would also pay a like charge, with the figure being set by hospital officials. The total revenue received was extremely important, since the hospital by law was required to be self-supporting.

In the early days of the Worcester hospital this system worked well; the state appropriation usually covered the costs of caring for state patients. By the early 1850s, however, hospital costs began to rise; in 1854 the state's contribution was below cost. The situation briefly improved, but the rapid inflation during the Civil War again widened the difference. The relative underpayment by the state, Jarvis pointed out, forced hospital authorities to make up the difference by increasing the rates charged to private patients. In other words, the hospital implicitly discriminated against private cases. Middle- and upper-lower-class groups were hardest hit by the turn of events, since they were not subsidized by either towns or the state and hence could not afford the cost of protracted confinement.

With income sufficient, but only sufficient, to meet the expenses of ordinary life, many of these families postpone, as long as possible, the dreaded day of increasing the drafts upon it; yet being accustomed to self-dependence for the supply of all their wants, they are unwilling to ask the aid of charity, and their natural and habitual self-respect, and perhaps their pride, forbid their applying to the town for assistance, and thus make their first confession of pauperism. They thus retain their deranged relative at home, from week to week, from month to month, and some from year to year.[42]

Surveying the policy of twenty-four other states, Jarvis pointed out that a number of them made far more generous provision for their insane population. Massachusetts, by way of contrast, discriminated against its native-born residents. "Our Irish patients go free and stay without cost, and they are sent early and have the best opportunities of restoration," he complained. "The Americans go at their own cost, and pay all and more than all of the expense of their support, and consequently a large proportion are kept away, some for months and years, as long as their friends can endure or take care of them, and many for life, because their friends lack courage or money to take due advantage of the means of restoration so largely provided in the State." Such a policy was costly, for the continued presence of insanity meant higher welfare costs. While not proposing full funding of mental hospitals by the state, Jarvis urged the legislature to alter the existing policy and grant the hospital sufficient operating funds.[43]

Nor did Jarvis confine his comments to economic issues. He condemned in strong language the practice of confining the criminally insane at the Worcester hospital, and urged the state to erect a separate institution for this class. Jarvis was equally critical of the relative absence of adequate occupational facilities for patients in public hospitals. His affirmation of the importance of occupational therapy had been reinforced two years earlier by his European experiences, and he insisted that the time had come for the state to provide sufficient facilities for the employment of all patients.[44]

For the next two years Jarvis continued his campaign to alter the manner in which the state financed its public hospitals. He began to lobby in the legislature and also sought the support of

Pliny Earle, a longtime colleague and superintendent of the Northampton hospital. Toward the end of 1864 he managed to persuade his fellow trustees to take the unusual step of submitting a memorial to the legislature. "It is a little remarkable," he wrote to Earle in an unsuccessful effort to convince the Northampton trustees to co-sponsor the petition, "that our State, instead of finding means to lighten the burden on the families of the poor or straitened circumstances should levy a heavy tax on them, when in the hospitals, by making them pay more than the actual cost, in order, that the Commonwealth may pay less for its patients, the Irish paupers!"[45]

In January 1865 the memorial was ready for submission to the general court. It repeated in detail Jarvis's earlier comments, and requested the commonwealth to pay for the entire cost of state paupers and to provide an appropriation of $2,000 to help defray the costs of supporting patients from families of limited means who could not afford to pay the total charges. Although all the trustees signed the petition, they were less than enthusiastic and provided minimal support at best; they saw no particular reason to engage in a conflict with the legislature. Nor did the newly created board of state charities endorse Jarvis's proposals; its report actually urged the legislature to authorize an increase in weekly payments for state paupers from $2.75 to $3.00. Jarvis was convinced that several officers of the board (excluding its president, Samuel Gridley Howe) had actively fought his proposal. In the end the legislature increased the weekly amount to $3.25. The basic dilemma, however, was left unresolved. Chronic financial problems continued to plague the hospital; a fixed sum did not take into account actual expenses or changes in the real value of money.[46] For Jarvis the results were particularly disheartening. State policy would continue to discriminate against families of moderate means with insane relatives. Ineligible for either local or state subsidies and unable to pay the costs of protracted care and treatment, such families would in all probability continue to avoid institutionalization.

Jarvis's unwillingness to assume a passive role introduced an element of discord into the board's deliberations. Although there were no open differences, it was clear that his presence was a disturbing element to those members unaccustomed to activism. Nor were state officials enamored with Jarvis, for during the 1860s Massachusetts was attempting to economize and retrench. Consequently, the governor did not reappoint Jarvis when his term on the board expired at the end of 1865—a most unusual action, since most state trustees generally retained their position as long as they were willing to serve.[47]

Given his temperament and personality, Jarvis could not restrict the scope of his activities to a single state. While fighting to change public policy within his native state, he also took part in national debates over a variety of policy issues. By then it was evident that the earlier promises of institutional care and treatment had not been fully realized. The rapid growth in the size of mental hospitals, the accumulation of seemingly incurable cases, the concern with managerial rather than therapeutic concerns, the growing pressure on hospitals from population increase, allegations that insane persons were being deprived of their civil rights, and the increase in welfare expenditures, all combined to give rise to a broad debate. None of these concerns were new to Jarvis; his *Report on Insanity* anticipated with remarkable acumen the problems of the future. Although removed from the sources of political power, Jarvis was not averse to contributing to the discussion of policy issues. Indeed, his self-image as an educator propelled him into the very midst of the discussions that were taking place within psychiatry and state legislatures.

Ultimately the debate revolved around several specific issues. Should separate custodial hospitals be established for chronic cases? To what degree could the British nonrestraint system be imposed in the United States? How could institutions provide more effective therapeutic care? Most important, what public policies were most appropriate for the care and treatment of the mentally ill.[48] Jarvis's contribution was less as a committed partisan and more as a sober intelligence disciplined by the available facts. Over sixty years of age and removed from the daily concerns of institutional psychiatrists, he assumed the mantle of an elder statesman. Unlike colleagues who omitted or ignored facts that did not fit their perceptions of reality or saw their opponents in conspiratorial terms, Jarvis's analyses were usually conditioned by the data that he had so meticulously collected for more than two decades. This is not in any way to imply that his ideological framework did not influence the manner in which he selected and interpreted his findings. It is only to say that Jarvis was somewhat more willing to acknowledge material that on occasion contradicted some of his deeply held convictions.

More so than the specialty at large, Jarvis's views were informed by his extensive knowledge of European practices. In 1860, for example, he prepared for the meetings of the Association of Medical Superintendents of American Institutions for the Insane a paper (read, in his absence, by a colleague) dealing with the advantages and desirability of private institutions or homes for the insane. Comparing England and America, he pointed out that the former had a dual system composed of public institutions for paupers and private establishments for persons of independent means. In the United States, however, most patients, private and public alike, were cared for in public hospitals. Conceding that the overwhelming majority of cases belonged in public institutions, he nevertheless envisaged a role for private hospitals or homes. Some insane persons were fearful of being stigmatized if the fact of their incarceration became public knowledge; others did not require the formal structure of large mental institutions. For both groups small private homes or hospitals served an important function by providing an environment ''resembling more nearly that of their own homes than can be offered and enjoyed in the public hospitals.''[49]

Jarvis's paper occasioned a lengthy and vigorous debate. A number of his colleagues conceded that small private hospitals or homes had a useful function, although proper classification would be impaired by lack of a sufficiently large number of patients. Those who were opposed to Jarvis's suggestion, however, saw no advantages whatsoever; they also feared that such institutions would be capable of abuse. Undoubtedly the growing public criticism of mental hospitals played a part in the lukewarm reception to Jarvis's paper. Most superintendents were of the opinion that the public or quasi-public nature of their institutions automatically limited abuses and hence provided a degree of protection against the charge that the rights of patients were often ignored. Jarvis's receptivity toward small private institutions, of course, mirrored his own experiences of having patients in his home or boarded nearby and under his supervision.[50]

One of the major issues confronting institutional psychiatry involved the use or nonuse of restraint. In some respects superintendents were caught on the horns of a dilemma. On the one hand, they were faced with certain forms of behavior that complicated the task of managing their hospitals in an efficient manner. Moreover, subtle but strong community pressure to prevent escapes by presumably dangerous patients implied greater security precautions within hospitals. On the other hand, there were critics who saw restraint as a violation of basic human rights and a substitute for therapy. They tended to favor the British nonrestraint system first popularized by John Conolly and Richard Gardner Hill in the 1840s.

The result was a bitter controversy that lasted for several decades. The overwhelming majority of American superintendents were opposed to the British system. Indeed, they charged their British brethren with a form of self-deception. Seclusion and isolation of patients in padded cells, techniques normally employed in England, in many instances adversely affected patients, Americans argued, since such practices removed them from virtually all human contact. And in cases where padded cells were not used, according to Isaac Ray, the English system was nothing more than bringing together "a great mass of patients of every description, under no restraint, and *taking their chance for the result.*" John Bull, he concluded, "like many other beasts is easily deceived by a little false show, especially when his self-complacency is gratified at the same time."[51]

To this debate Jarvis brought a somewhat different perspective, in part an outgrowth of his European observations in 1860. Americans, he told Thomas S. Kirkbride (author of the influential *On the Construction, Organization, and General Arrangements of Hospitals for the Insane* [1854]), had much to learn from their foreign counterparts. English and European hospitals employed about eighty percent of their patients, thereby diminishing the need for restraint. Indeed, these institutions had "no strong rooms, no means of confining hand or arm or foot.

Neither camisoles. Straps are abolished. Some of the asylums have no grated or iron-protected windows." In Jarvis's eyes, therefore, the problem was less one of restraint versus nonrestraint and more one of providing sufficient occupational facilities for all patients.[52]

In 1862 Jarvis summed up his views in a controversial paper at the Association of Medical Superintendents convention. The most striking feature of English hospitals, he noted, was "the quietness and loneliness of the wards during the daytime." Rather than moping aimlessly about, virtually all patients were employed in a variety of occupations. Indeed, no new institution was built in England without including appropriate occupational facilities. But above all, meaningful labor, apart from any economic benefits, was an important therapeutic tool. In closing Jarvis urged his colleagues to follow the British example, thereby offering to curable patients "a faculty of restoration" and to incurable ones a "means of diminishing their morbid excitability and distress and of lessening the burden of their disease."[53]

Jarvis's comments touched a sensitive nerve among colleagues, if only because of the implication that American hospitals were not the equal of their British counterparts. John Curwen and Isaac Ray implicitly conceded the accuracy of Jarvis's observations by placing responsibility for the absence of labor upon the character of patients and the nature of the American social structure. Curwen maintained that American patients were more excited and often refused to work since their board was already paid. Moreover, the quality of the attendant corps precluded the adoption of an effective system. Ray also argued that a deferential society in England made patients more amenable to work. Systematic labor, he added, implied less supervision and greater opportunities for escape. British patients who found a higher standard of living within institutions were less prone to take advantage of their relative freedom, whereas Americans, many of whom held higher expectations, would not be as restrained. Even those who did not markedly disagree with Jarvis's general analysis insisted that lack of facilities precluded following the British example. Jarvis's response was unequivocal: if labor was of therapeutic value, facilities should be made available.

Indeed, as a trustee of the Worcester hospital, he launched a campaign to provide adequate occupational opportunities for as many patients as possible.[54]

Within a few years Jarvis was drawn into another national controversy that had its origins in the overcrowded conditions at most public mental hospitals and the accumulation of chronic patients. Massachusetts already recognized the problem when it established in the late 1850s a separate department for incurably insane paupers at one of its state almshouses. The action of the New York legislature in accepting the recommendation of Sylvester Willard to establish a central public institution for incurable patients set off a fierce controversy that threatened to split the young specialty. The Association of Medical Superintendents, which represented the views of the founders of institutional psychiatry, took a decidedly negative stance; it remained unalterably opposed to institutions for incurable persons. Its members refused to modify their faith in the curability of mental disease; the basic issue in their eyes was the size of hospitals and the availability of sufficient resources for the fulfillment of a therapeutic mission. Their critics, on the other hand, felt that more efficient and economical modes of care were desirable and possible, particularly since many individuals failed to recover in more costly therapeutic institutions.[55]

As an elder statesman, Jarvis could not remain aloof. His earlier work on the relationship between distance from a hospital and frequency of use was well known. It was not surprising, therefore, that a committee of the New York legislature sought Jarvis's counsel. The result was a report to the legislature (published in the *American Journal of Insanity*) that updated his earlier findings. Unlike colleagues who continued to debate the merits of curable and incurable institutions, Jarvis chose to put the issue in an entirely different light. The decision, he insisted, was simply between another large hospital serving the adjacent population or three smaller ones geographically dispersed in the western, northeastern, and southeastern parts of the state.[56]

Although Jarvis's contribution to the debate was sober and informed, his views were generally ignored. Most superintendents were preoccupied with other concerns and were unable to incorporate such findings into their outlook. The legislature, by way of contrast, tended to define the issue in terms of economy and efficiency; its members had no institutional mechanism capable of assimilating data to policy. Moreover, Jarvis's dispassionate presentation lacked the emotional content characteristic of the debate. In the end his views went unheeded and the legislature authorized the establishment of a large institution for chronic cases.[57]

V

As a physician who defined his role in preventive terms, Jarvis on occasion became peripherally involved in some of the moral issues that agitated American politics in the nineteenth century. Since his youthful days in Concord he had remained convinced that the use of alcohol had pernicious effects upon health. Yet he was never active in the temperance or prohibition movements, partly because they were secondary to his primary concerns. Nevertheless, the aggregate data he collected only reinforced his belief that alcohol and mortality were related. In 1864 he prepared a study of the ''effect of intemperance upon life'' for Governor Andrew in the hope of influencing policy. Two years later he published a brief article in the *Boston Medical and Surgical Journal* in which he employed statistical data to demonstrate a causal relationship between disease, mortality, and intemperance. Although the anti-liquor tone of the article was self-evident, it proposed no specific remedies or policies.[58]

In early 1867 the liquor question was thrust into state politics when the legislature was presented with a petition, bearing nearly 35,000 signatures, requesting passage of a licensing law in place of the existing prohibitory law enacted more than a decade before. The anti-liquor forces in turn presented petitions with an even larger number of signatures, and the stage was set for a bitter political debate over an issue that aroused passions on all sides. The leadership of the movement to enact a licensing law was assumed by former Governor Andrew, who attempted to refute the prohibitionist claims about the poisonous character of alcohol and its supposed relationship to immoral and criminal behavior.[59]

The prohibitionist forces, led by the Rev. A.A. Miner (president of Tufts College) called a number of witnesses before a special joint committee of the legislature, including Jarvis. In his testimony Jarvis attempted to demonstrate the deletorious effects that followed the use of alcohol. To buttress his case he cited as authorities Benedict A. Morel's *Traités des degénérescences, physiques, intellectuales et morales de l'espèce humaine et des causes qui produisent ces variétés maladives* (1857) and F.G.P. Nieson's *Contributions to Vital Statistics* (1857). Jarvis's testimony was cut short by the lateness of the hour; there was no opportunity for the opposing side to conduct a cross-examination.[60]

In presenting the argument for licensing, Andrew attempted to demonstrate that the so-called statistics were at best judgments that reflected individual biases. He singled out Jarvis's testimony, if only because the latter's reputation as a statistician and an individual disassociated from partisanship could prove damaging. Alluding to the fact that Jarvis had not been subjected to cross-examination, Andrew tried to refute the statistical evidence by showing that Morel's work was founded on too small a sample, and that a good deal of Jarvis's data and interpretations were erroneous.[61]

Andrew's attack angered Jarvis, partly because misuse of evidence represented an unforgiveable sin. In this respect his behavior was consistent; he also wrote to Miner to condemn the manner in which the prohibitionist forces misquoted Morel and the mortality census that had recently been published by the federal government. The brunt of his anger, however, was directed toward Andrew, who had extended Jarvis's statements beyond their original meaning. The comparison of states by the use of data from mental hospital reports, for example, was completely unjustified, if only because hospital statistics bearing on the relationship between insanity and intemperance were not necessarily representative of the state in which the institution was located. Moreover, Jarvis specifically pointed out that his citation of census mortality statistics was explicitly qualified by a statement that the returns were imperfect. In dismissing Andrew's charges, Jarvis concluded that "it is the right & the duty of the body politic & the government, to try every means within its power to prevent their use; & I see no better way to effect this than by a prohibitory law." Such a statement, of course, conflicted in part with his faith in education and voluntaristic ideology. Yet Jarvis remained unaware of this contradiction. His distaste for alcohol led him to insist, as he told Miner, "that it is the duty of the government to use all its power to extinguish this enemy in the midst of our people."[62]

VI

In some cases advancing age is accompanied by a disillusionment with the present and a romanticization of the past. In Jarvis's case this generalization does not apply. As he grew older, his faith in the reality and possibility of progress remained as firm as ever. Although retaining a sentimental remembrance of his beloved Concord, he never compared the present unfavorably with the past. Indeed, during a lengthy debate at the meetings of the Association of Medical Superintendents of American Institutions for the Insane in 1862, he explicitly rejected the widely held proposition that the advance of civilization brought in its wake a disproportionate increase in the incidence of insanity. "Wherever and whenever population increases, as it has in this country and in almost every civilized nation," he told his colleagues, "there has been, and there will be, an increase of the number of the insane, at least in the same proportion, unless the causes which produce insanity are arrested. If these are constant, their effects, the disordered brains, must be constant. And whatever variation there may be in the number and proportion of the insane, for the increase or for the decrease, it is owing to a preceding variation in the extent and force of the causes." When queried by Isaac Ray, Jarvis denied that modern civilization had diminished man's vital power or decreased longevity; the very opposite was true.[63] The continued existence of social evils was not a sufficient reason to despair. On the contrary, it provided mankind with an opportunity to apply reason and science and thus forge a better world. And Jarvis never for a moment doubted the possibility of human improvement. Failures were not a product of immutable human frailties; he had no patience with Calvinism or a view of a species forever stained by original sin.

In 1869 he summed up his lifelong faith in progress in a long peroration in the *Atlantic Monthly*. Noting the constant allusions to the degeneracy of contemporary society, he nevertheless dismissed them. "The same was said last year and in the last century," he told his readers. "Looking through the records of many hundred years past, we find, in every age, the same complaints, the same sorrowful discontent with the present, the same hopeless distrust of the future, and the same respect for the past." All such claims about human degeneracy, however, were demonstrably false. Indeed, the quality and quantity of life, if anything, were increasing rather than decreasing; people lived longer and enjoyed better health. In modern society there was less destitution than previously, and the "growth of charity and mutual love and respect" tempered the preoccupation with brute force so characteristic of earlier ages. "Although civilization has done so much for human life, it has not yet wrought its perfect work," Jarvis concluded.

How long it will take to complete this work of human development and longevity,—how many generations must pass before threescore and ten years, instead of being the maximum as the psalmist thought, and the lot of only the favored and the few as now, will be the minimum, the assured lot of all the children of men,—we cannot tell, nor is it needful for us to know. Sufficient for us is it to know that, by carefulness and culture, life has increased, and to feel assured that by the same means it may be still further increased; and as we received a richer legacy of life from our fathers than they received from theirs, so it is our duty and our privilege to improve this heritage, to add our part to its worth and its power, and leave it to our children more effective and enduring than we found it.[64]

8

Modernizing the Federal Census

Jarvis's varied activities during the early and mid-1860s were so intense that they might have taxed the energies of younger men. His commitment to social improvement, however, proved a constant stimulant. When the eighth census entered the planning phase, therefore, Jarvis leaped at the opportunity to influence its structure and organization. Familiar with the limitations of the census, he remained as determined as ever to make certain that the mistakes of the past were not repeated. His first opportunity came when he was asked to prepare the volume dealing with the mortality statistics, a task he undertook with enthusiasm. When Representative James A. Garfield sought his advice about drafting legislation to create a more accurate census in 1869, Jarvis was again delighted to be of assistance. His involvement ultimately helped to pave the way for the creation of the modern federal census.

I

In early 1859 the federal government began to make preparations for the eighth census. Much to the surprise of some, the new census was modeled after its predecessor. Under the act of May 23, 1850, the secretary of the interior was empowered to take future censuses along the lines stipulated in the law if Congress did not enact new legislation before January 1 of the year in which a census was supposed to be taken. Since Congress had not acted, the secretary of the interior simply followed the procedures mandated a decade earlier. Joseph C.G. Kennedy was appointed superintendent, and the same schedules used in 1850 (with a few minor modifications) were printed.

In the spring of 1859 the American Statistical Association authorized Jarvis to prepare a memorial dealing with the census, which was sent to the secretary of the interior in August. At the same time Jarvis wrote to Kennedy and spelled out in detail specific shortcomings of the previous census. Still concerned with the mortality statistics, he urged Kennedy to obtain information on all of the *births* (as well as the deaths) that occurred between June 1, 1859, and June 1, 1860. It could not be assumed that children age one or less and alive at the end of the year represented the number of births in that period (as Congress had assumed a decade earlier in the legislation providing for the taking of the census). Finally, he requested once again that the errors in the census of 1840 be corrected, since such data was still being used by those unaware of their deficiencies.[1]

Kennedy's reply was noncommital. Jarvis then suggested that the secretary of the interior interpret the law in a liberal manner and assume that he had the power to do everything that was not explicitly forbidden. In another communication Jarvis pointed out that the manuscript mortality returns provided the potential to present "a popular nosology or nomenclature of diseases . . . especially as connected with localities." The returns could then be worked over by competent medical authorities and the result would be a nosology that went far beyond anything then available.[2]

Jarvis heard nothing further from Kennedy during the spring and summer of 1860. But in September Jarvis received a communication from James Wynne, who was also seeking to have the preparation of the mortality statistics placed under the direction of a qualified physician. Wynne had written to Kennedy and proposed that he and Jarvis collaborate in preparing the mortality statistics. Kennedy responded by requesting a detailed plan, whereupon Wynne wrote to Jarvis. Within a month Jarvis sent Wynne a proposal of over forty pages that summarized all of the changes he had been urging for nearly a decade.[3]

Jarvis, however, was not sanguine about the possibility of having his plan adopted. The federal government, unlike its counterparts in England and Western Europe, was not in the habit of having scientific work "executed by scientific men," he wrote to Wynne. Indeed, the government's refusal to compensate him for his labor on the seventh census was indicative of the attitudes of public officials generally. His fears were not without some foundation. During a meeting in Washington, Wynne presented to Kennedy a plan based largely on Jarvis's letter. Claiming to detect a note of hostility in Kennedy's attitude toward Jarvis, Wynne then proposed turning the preparation of the mortality statistics over to himself, since he intended to seek Jarvis's aid and to share the compensation. Although Kennedy's initial attitude seemed favorable, he eventually selected Dr. Josiah Curtis, a Massachusetts physician noted for his interest in public health and registration, to work on the mortality statistics. Kennedy, complained Wynne, was simply a "politician."[4] The selection of Curtis momentarily aborted Jarvis's desire to play a major role in the preparation of the mortality volume.

For nearly two years Jarvis heard nothing further. The outbreak of the Civil War had a disastrous effect upon this project. The work on the mortality statistics came to a virtual halt when Curtis resigned from the census department to join the Union Army in the fall of 1861, although the census office continued to aggregate the manuscript returns. In May 1862 Kennedy sent a preliminary report to Congress, in which he described with pride the continued growth of the nation's population. In his summary of the mortality figures Kennedy conceded that the total number of deaths in the census was grossly inaccurate; he estimated that the actual number of deaths during the twelve months following June 1, 1859, was about 680,000 (as compared with the reported number of 392,821).[5]

Nevertheless, the *Preliminary Report* was not without its problems. Kennedy, Jarvis wrote to a friend a few years later, admitted that the volume was "hastily written and imperfectly digested." Many of his aides were "merely politicians . . . whose mental habits were undisciplined." The only redeeming hope was that the final volumes would correct the errors perpetuated in the initial report.[6]

Recognizing the necessity of securing the services of competent and knowledgeable individuals, Kennedy approached Jarvis in the spring of 1863. At a meeting in Washington the two came to a quick agreement. Jarvis was given the task of preparing the commentary or philosophical part of the mortality report, which would be based on the raw material supplied by Kennedy. It was also agreed that Jarvis would have maximum freedom and considerable discretionary authority. Compensation was set at $1,800 per year, and additional funds would be made available for clerical help. To Jarvis the importance of the project completely overshadowed the relatively low rate of compensation. Nor did his private practice interpose a barrier, for his wife's health now made it difficult to accept private patients in his home.[7]

As the raw materials arrived from Washington during the spring and summer of 1863, Jarvis's worst fears about their reliability were confirmed. Internal contradictions abounded; the number of deaths from yellow fever in Pennsylvania was larger than the total for the country as a whole. Other discrepancies were more serious. The census of 1850, for example, listed a total of 276,088 male slaves under the age of five. The figure for this same group in 1860 (age ten to fifteen) was 276,711. Given the high death rate among young children generally, it was clear that the total for 1860 had to be substantially less than the figures for the preceding decade. Although Jarvis was inclined to attribute the errors to underreporting in 1850, it was evident that the quality of the data posed major difficulties. A similar discrepancy appeared in the figures for the native-born white population.[8]

Even more distressing was the fact that the mortality data sent to Jarvis made no distinctions as to country of birth or color. "It will be important," he informed Kennedy in requesting that the census office reaggregate the returns in its possession, "to show the mortality of the blacks, mulattoes & whites separately, & also of natives & foreigners." The susceptibility of whites and blacks to disease and their liability to death varied so greatly "that a mixture of the two would vitiate any comparison of this country with any other, in respect to disease and mortality." Finally, the data on immigrants and their children also presented formidable obstacles. The reports of arrivals in the United States were not complete; they did not provide a reliable age distribution (with the exception of those under forty); and they did not distinguish between returning Americans and foreigners visiting the United States. The failure of the census to distinguish between children of immigrant and native-born parents compounded the problems of an admittedly inadequate data base.[9]

Disheartened by the shortcomings in the raw data, Jarvis spent nearly two years attempting to convince Kennedy to have his clerks reaggregate the original returns into separate categories for white and black, and immigrant and native born. Like many Americans, Jarvis assumed a relationship between social and medical problems on the one hand and ethnicity and race on the other; the categories he proposed for the census schedules merely reflected this perception. Consequently, his request to have immigrants and blacks reported separately was not accompanied by a corresponding appeal to have the population broken down by income-distribution categories. Yet he did not necessarily draw invidious conclusions about immigrants or blacks. His search for knowledge reflected a desire to aid in the task of improving the health of all segments of society. Others were less cautious than Jarvis, and they did not hesitate to attribute to minority ethnic and racial groups responsibility for pressing social problems.[10]

Jarvis initially sent to Kennedy a copy of the original plan that he had drawn up for Wynne in 1860. This plan required that the data be reaggregated in Washington. Much to Jarvis's regret, his suggestions for an ambitious analysis of the mortality data went unheeded. In 1864, therefore, he offered a more modest proposal.[11] By 1865, however, it was clear that Jarvis's proposals were doomed. The final decision came as no surprise. Indeed, Jarvis had already anticipated the outcome, relying in his own work upon estimates and hypothetical calculations. He also launched a major effort to add to his collection of foreign and domestic statistical reports in the hope of improving the quality of the data. In fact, he sought to secure copies of life tables from insurance companies that purportedly provided coverage for slaves.[12]

Deciding to make the best of a bad situation, Jarvis began to work out alternative means of estimating differential mortality patterns for immigrants and blacks. A detailed breakdown of immigrants was not available, although the seventh and eighth

censuses had listed the number of each sex of this group in the
United States in 1850 and 1860. By extrapolating from the Irish
immigration reports (a group that accounted for slightly more
than half of all arriving foreigners between 1850 and 1860) and
also working out a method of allowing for American and foreign
travelers, Jarvis arrived at an estimate of the number of immigrants arriving during the decade of the 1850s as well as their
age distribution. He then estimated probable mortality rates
among this group by using a combination of a logarithmic
method and by applying existing English and Irish life tables.
These procedures necessitated nearly five hundred separate com-
putations, but the result in his eyes was an accurate approxima-
tion of the number of foreign-born and their mortality in 1860.[13]

Jarvis also attempted to demonstrate the existence of an important differential between black and white mortality rates although the data base was even worse than that dealing with
immigrants. All the evidence, however, seemed to confirm a
differential rate, including data for white soldiers and native
blacks in the British West Indies. Conceding that "difference in
social & domestic condition" might play a role, he thought it
likely that "differences of constitution" were more important.
Moreover, climate was a variable that affected the races in different ways, for "cold is more fatal to the blacks & the heat more
fatal to whites." But as long as the two races were aggregated together, "no clear statement" could be made nor any "satisfac-
tory inference drawn, as to the morbidic & mortuary influences
of any climate or country." Were a separate record for each race
available, he advised Kennedy, "we should have a clear basis for
comparing the Caucasian race of this country in respect to their
diseases & deaths, & thereby approximately determine the climatic, terrestrial, endemic or other influences on the health &
life of the people of the United States."[14]

The two years following 1863 were particularly frustrating to
Jarvis because all of his proposals were ignored or rejected. Only
the fact that the federal government was involved in a bloody
war tempered the intensity of his feelings. By the spring of 1865,
however, the war finally ended. But at precisely this time Congress, probably because of an oversight, failed to pass an appropriation for the census department. The secretary of the interior

then dissolved the department and transferred its functions to the General Land Office. Jarvis, of course, was disappointed on several counts. Although he never said so in explicit terms, perhaps his greatest disappointment was the inability or reluctance of the federal government to recognize the intrinsic importance of the census as a source of knowledge and an instrument of policy. "Very few," he noted in 1867 while recounting his involvement with the eighth census, "have any conception of the looseness of many of our public reports and the care that is needed to correct or compensate for their error."[15]

During the spring of 1865 Jarvis was in touch with James Harlan, the secretary of the interior. Harlan was anxious to have the final census volume, including the mortality part, ready for Congress when it met toward the end of 1865. After meeting with Jarvis and receiving a memo outlining a plan for the mortality section, Harlan concluded an agreement whereby Jarvis would remain in Massachusetts and be authorized to hire a sufficient number of clerks to complete the project. During the summer and fall Jarvis worked frantically to complete the project while avoiding some of the gross errors that appeared in earlier census volumes. But the raw material sent from Washington contained errors and inconsistencies. A close examination revealed that the number of people who had died from each disease in the several states did not correspond with the total number stated to have died in the same states or to the total number of deaths due to the same disease when arranged according to the time of death. In other cases children were reported to have died of old age and older people of childhood diseases such as teething. There were other obvious errors. Upon encountering such anomalies, Jarvis used his own judgment to correct the figures as best he could.[16]

Although time did not permit consultations with other sanitarians or statisticians, Jarvis did send a preliminary table of contents to Edwin M. Snow, the distinguished sanitarian. Snow approved of the preliminary outline but feared that Jarvis would be unable to stay within his proposed limits. Much more important were the deficiencies in the data compiled from the manuscript census returns. It was possible to utilize data from the registration reports from states like Rhode Island and Massachusetts, but to compare these two states with others whose figures were far more unreliable was a dangerous procedure. Snow also expressed grave reservations about comparing mortality rates of foreigners and native-born persons, for the data did not distinguish between children of native-born and foreign parents (thus vitiating the validity of comparisons).[17]

At the end of October Jarvis sent to Washington the first installment of the mortality volume, which included ten tables and 228 manuscript pages. He may have hoped that Harlan would grant him additional time for a more detailed and sophisticated analysis. His hopes proved to be ill-founded; Harlan was determined to have the completed work in the hands of Congress by December. On November 18 Jarvis bowed to Harlan's wishes and all but surrendered any lingering hope that the mortality section might provide the government with an "opportunity to teach these lessons of human life, its powers & its dangers, to the people." By December the work was substantially complete, with the exception of the preface, the final reading of proof, and the preparation of a separate index. A few months later the final volume of the eighth census was published.[18]

The mortality statistics, which comprised nearly half of the six-hundred-page volume, were divided into two distinct parts. The first was a general forty-four page Introduction that included a series of summary tables; the second was the aggregated raw data presented in forty-eight tables with accompanying explanations. In the Introduction Jarvis summarized the data findings, offered some generalizations, and specified the limitations of the census. The report, he admitted on the first page, was "far from being as complete as desirable, because the primary bases on which it rests are imperfect." The mortality census, Jarvis concluded, "affords no opportunity of determining the reliable rate of mortality in the country . . . [and] it fails to teach some of the most important lessons which it was hoped might be derived from it."[19]

This did not mean, he added, that the mortality figures were worthless. By assuming that the reported deaths "fell in the same proportion on males and on females, happened in the same proportion in the several months, and from the same proportions of the several causes, and took away the same proportion of the several ages," it was possible to compare the health of people in different areas by using death as a criteria. Given the fact that the census office had not abstracted mortality by color or race, it was impossible to distinguish between the races. Other forms of evidence, however, indicated that race and country of birth played an important role in differential mortality rates.[20]

Jarvis then went on to describe the nosological system and defined nine geographical areas in terms of their climate and population composition. What Jarvis was seeking to convey was the idea that there were a number of complex variables that affected morbidity and mortality patterns; he feared that erroneous conclusions might be drawn by individuals who were unsophisticated in statistical techniques or by others who hoped to use the data to support their ideological prejudices.[21]

Jarvis's concern with a more accurate census was especially evident in his analysis of the political and economic consequences of population growth, both in the present and future. Society, he noted, was composed of dependent (young and old) and self-sustaining groups. The power of the population at any given time was simply the ratio "which the sustaining and dependent classes bear to each other," whereas the nation's future power would be in proportion to the numbers in the formative stages of growth. The American people therefore had a vested interest in understanding the conditions of health in different geographical regions, for this factor, in part, would determine the proportion of those surviving the vicissitudes of infancy and childhood and becoming part of the sustaining class. The nation's future well-being obviously rested to some degree on the ratio of the two classes.[22]

In the final section of the Introduction Jarvis provided some summary data dealing with the impact of immigration and patterns of internal migration. A knowledge of these social movements was important, for "if the record could be obtained, it would show how far the human constitution is capable of change of external condition, and whether one's native climate is the only one he can bear and sustain his strength unimpaired." What was perhaps most notable about this section was Jarvis's dispassionate analysis, which avoided invidious conclusions about the purported superiority of native-born as compared with immigrants; his discussion of the data throughout this section was neutral and impartial in tone.[23]

Jarvis's Introduction reflected both his own intellectual and scientific commitments as well as the deadline within which he was working. He deliberately refused to offer any final generalizations about the conditions of health, morbidity, and mortality, and stressed instead the limitations of the census findings. "I do not like to go to the world with any doctrine until I have *all* proof that the subject admits," he wrote to a colleague early in 1868. "In my report of mortality . . . I especially disclaimed all these inferences & cautioned people against them, as they lead to error in respect to health & mortality of the States & the country."[24] In the statistical section that followed his Introduction, Jarvis presented the census returns in a variety of forms.[25]

In terms of statistical methodology Jarvis was no innovator. His conception and knowledge of statistics, compared with some contemporaries, were relatively rudimentary. Nor was he especially well-versed in either political economy or mathematics, which were beginning to merge with the growing body of statistical data and give rise to a method that ultimately became the basis for social science and social medicine. Moreover, Jarvis was not cognizant of the problems inherent in collecting unbiased observations or of deciding when the number of observations was large enough to be a representative sample, to say nothing about making classification the basis of science.[26] In this respect he was not unique; a good part of the medical statistics of the mid-nineteenth century reflected the fusion or religious and moral concepts with a Baconian view of science.

II

By the time the eighth census was completed, the time for taking the ninth was already approaching. As matters stood, the framework for preparing the new census would remain unchanged unless Congress enacted new legislation to supersede the law of May 23, 1850. Early in 1869 James A. Garfield, then a member of the House of Representatives, emerged as the leading member of the Committee on the Ninth Census. Aware of the shortcomings of earlier enumerations, Garfield wanted Congress to enact legislation that would reorganize completely both the taking and compiling of the census. In his eyes legislation required a thorough knowledge of reality, and reality was most easily expressed in statistical terms. "This is an age of statistics," proclaimed Garfield in words that would have met with an enthusiastic approval by Jarvis.[27]

Some months earlier Garfield began to solicit the names of individuals who were qualified to provide him with advice and assistance in preparing such legislation. Henry Villard, secretary of the American Social Science Association in Boston, immediately recommended Jarvis. "That he is an authority well worth consulting," Villard wrote Garfield, "appears from the fact, that he furnished the ground plan for the census of 1850."[28]

Accepting Villard's advice, Garfield contacted Jarvis, as well as several other prominent figures. Garfield was especially concerned with the manner in which the census would be taken as well as the type of data collected.[29] Within two weeks Jarvis had prepared a lengthy communication in which he spelled out his views regarding the personnel to be employed, the procedures to be followed, and suggestions for revising existing schedules. The eighth census, he added, could have contained more analytic material if federal officials had been more patient and allowed sufficient time for reflection.[30]

Two days later Jarvis sent Garfield a second communication that dealt with some general problems. Citing earlier deficiencies, Jarvis blamed the personnel employed in the field and in Washington.[31] On March 1 he sent Garfield two additional letters. The first made two suggestions: the American government should investigate the British and Irish censuses; and the new enumeration should distinguish between blacks and mulattoes. The second offered specific illustrations of errors in earlier federal censuses in order to underscore the need for qualified staff. Jarvis's letters received an enthusiastic reception from Garfield, who shared a fear that the accuracy of the census might be fatally impaired if political appointees were once again employed. Indeed, Garfield ordered three of the letters printed for the use of his committee.[32]

If Garfield was pleased with Jarvis's responses, others had reservations. Dr. Franklin B. Hough, the former superintendent of the New York State and District of Columbia censuses and an avowed candidate for the superintendency of the ninth census, was dubious about some of Jarvis's proposals. Hough thought it impossible to take the census within a single day; he disagreed with the use of tax assessors as enumerators, fearing that people would interpret the questions as heralding a new tax and therefore be disinclined to provide accurate answers; and he was critical of Jarvis's emphasis on the importance of an accurate nosology on the grounds that most people could not identify a specific disease. Hough, as a matter of fact, felt that a census was "but a meagre and miserable substitute for a Registration System, and [no] *census* [could] ever meet the strict demands of science in this particular."[33]

By the end of March Garfield's committee was far enough along in its work to introduce a comprehensive bill to reorganize the federal census. The bill proposed that a census bureau be created in the Interior Department under a superintendent nominated by the President and confirmed by the Senate. Each congressional district would have an assistant superintendent, who would employ sufficient enumerators to take the census within a month. After amendments substantially altered the original bill, Garfield accepted a resolution calling for the appointment of a special committee to report by the end of the year.[34]

Garfield and the new committee shortly thereafter began to prepare a new bill and drafts of census schedules. During May and June, Garfield called upon a number of individuals for assistance. Among them was Jarvis, who agreed to prepare a plan to collect accurate population statistics and then to testify before the full committee in June. Immediately following his appearance in Washington, Jarvis attended the convention of the Association of Medical Superintendents in Virginia, where he asked the delegates to cooperate in filling out the schedule dealing with patients. When some hesitation was expressed about violating confidentiality, Jarvis assured his colleagues that the purpose was not to make the names of individuals public, but rather to prevent repetition.[35]

At the end of June the committee adjourned. Hough (who was employed on a temporary basis by Garfield) was pessimistic about the future, partly because the committee was divided on the issue of recommending a more permanent census office. He also feared that the marshalls ("who would be deprived of a profitable job by a change of the law"), together with other allies, would either delay congressional action or else mutilate the bill in order to forestall changes. "I will however say," he wrote to Jarvis, "and in this *I know you will agree with me:* that a government work, and especially one on which so many useful interests depend as on the census, should be, both *in fact and in appearance,* entirely free from taint, *of private interests,* as well as from those that tend to serve *sectional, partisan* or *private objects, individual theories, or selfish ends.*" To put it another way, Hough was implying that an effective census was one of the few instruments capable of serving as a mediator between science and policy and thereby eliminating political and partisan considerations from the policy-making process.[36]

During the remainder of 1869 Jarvis continued to serve as a paid consultant. In December Garfield submitted the final version of his bill to Congress together with a lengthy report. Tracing the history of the census since ancient times, Garfield's report defended census reform. He also included in an appendix a document prepared by Jarvis that constituted about one-fifth of the report. Jarvis's paper spelled out in summary form his mature views on the subject. The bill, Garfield privately admitted, fell far short of what he and Jarvis desired, "but the constant danger of overloading it by attempting too much, prevented us from enlarging its scope." Jarvis, nevertheless, was pleased with Garfield's work, particularly since the bill incorporated many of his own recommendations.[37]

After a lengthy debate the bill passed the House by a vote of 86 to 40. Under its provisions the census would be taken in one month; enumerators would be chosen for every congressional district and compensated on a per diem basis. But in the Senate the bill encountered formidable opposition. In Garfield's eyes the issue of patronage was paramount. "A desire to retain the Marshalls and thus retain the patronage in their hands seems to be the motive that influences many Senators," he remarked. No doubt the fact that the opposition was led by Roscoe Conkling of New York seemed to lend credence to Garfield's charge.[38]

On the other hand, there were some who were persuaded that the House bill represented no improvement whatsoever. Edwin M. Snow in particular thought Garfield's proposal "cumbersome and expensive, and absolutely impracticable." "I also condemned the previous schedule section," he added in a letter to Jarvis, "on account of expense far beyond benefit, though I would like to see the experiment tried in a cheaper way." Snow eventually came to the conclusion that the ninth census would be better taken under the existing statute, especially if Francis Amasa Walker, the newly appointed superintendent of the census, remained in office. Snow preferred that Congress pass a general law specifying the machinery and objectives of the census, but leaving its implementation to the superintendent. The fact that time was growing short was another important consideration. "Personally," Snow wrote to Garfield in mid-January, "I very much regretted to be obliged to differ from your matured opinions upon the subject . . . but being so firmly convinced of the correctness of my views, I could not avoid it. I think your bill was very much injured by the additions and amendments. . . . At any rate, I hope you will believe I had no object in view, but the best good of the census." Snow's opposition had a powerful effect on the Senate. Kennedy in addition rejected allegations that the seventh and eighth censuses were inadequate. Although Jarvis did what little he could to rally support in the Senate, his efforts proved futile. On February 9, 1870, the Senate rejected the House bill by the overwhelming vote of 47 to 9.[39]

Shortly thereafter Congress enacted a slightly modified version of the act of May 23, 1850. For Garfield the bill was a bitter pill to swallow. Jarvis was equally distressed at the outcome. The fact that the debate had not touched upon the merits of the House bill only exacerbated his annoyance. Ultimately, he concluded, "a cheap census, its errors & imperfections, is a very costly matter to the country."[40]

Only the knowledge that the ninth census would be supervised by Walker mitigated Jarvis's bitterness. When defeat seemed imminent, Jarvis immediately wrote to Walker and repeated many of his former suggestions. Toward the end of 1871 Jarvis received the initial volumes of the ninth census, which contained the population and vital statistics. Although impressed with their clarity, Jarvis thought that another opportunity to contribute to human knowledge had once again been lost. Walker had not distinguished between white-black or native-immigrant mortality, thus rendering impossible the task of discriminating between the health and vitality of the races. An improvement over its predecessors, the ninth census nevertheless fell far short of Jarvis's expectations or hopes.[41] Walker himself was cognizant of many of the shortcomings of the census; he estimated that as much as 40 percent of the actual deaths were unreported.[42]

III

After 1870 Jarvis's involvement with the federal census came to an end.[43] By the time the tenth census was taken a decade later, he was nearly eighty years old and the infirmities of age had taken their toll. What can be said, in summary, about Jarvis's contributions to the census? If he had not succeeded in achieving his goal of making the census a body of authoritative data that could be used to illuminate the conditions of health, he at least had added significantly to the growing awareness of its defects and its potentialities. When he first became aware of the inadequacies of the federal census in 1842, there was relatively little concern about its validity. To most the census served simply to determine political representation or as a source of national pride. By the 1870s, on the other hand, the potentialities of the census were more fully recognized. More and more researchers shared Jarvis's faith in the census as an instrument that would illuminate certain social problems that threatened the very fabric of the nation and would end once and for all needless political conflict over policy issues.

In Jarvis's philosophy, accurate data would help to bring

about the creation of a moral and prosperous society. It was in-conceivable that valid knowledge could in any way be put to im-moral uses. A firm believer in progress, he looked forward to a time when an educated and enlightened society would fully em-ploy its wisdom and knowledge to resolve its problems and create a virtuous and just social order. Similarly, he saw in the census the means whereby the medical profession could finally fulfil its promise by offering a definitive analysis of the individ-ual and environmental origins of disease.

Curiously enough, the creation of the census in its modern form in 1880 and 1890 came precisely at a time when the charac-ter of the medical profession had so changed that physicians like Jarvis seemed a relic of a bygone age. By then the belief that dis-ease was a consequence of an improper environment and indi-vidual misbehavior was partially succeeded by the germ theory and its identification of microscopic organisms with specific dis-ease entities. The goal of medicine correspondingly shifted from the prevention of disease through environmental controls to the identification and eradication of specific diseases through medical and scientific intervention. Within this newer tradition the need for an elaborate taxonomy and quantified data dimin-ished sharply; the well-equipped laboratory and hospital with their pathological and bacteriological research facilities assumed a paramount position. Jarvis, however, was oblivious to the in-tellectual and scientific changes that were radically transforming the medical profession. Having grown to maturity in a different age, his view of medicine was inseparably linked with a set of particular moral and scientific assumptions that gave coherence to his concepts of health and disease. Paradoxically, his concern with the census was to be taken up not by the medical profes-sion, but by the emerging social and behavioral sciences which were destined to use quantification and statistics along the lines foreseen by Jarvis. In so doing, the social and behavioral sciences would also inherit the dilemmas inherent in any scientific system based upon taxonomical principles.

9
Twilight

In the quarter of a century following the end of the Civil War, medicine underwent a series of changes that ultimately transformed theory and practice. Slowly but surely its habitat became the laboratory rather than society; bacteriology and cellular pathology replaced broad statistical investigation. The result was a sharp definition of medical roles. To Jarvis, who represented the older tradition, the proper function of the physician was to act "as a prophylactic adviser to warn the people of danger and keep them in the path of health."[1] Ultimate responsibility for maintaining health and preventing disease, however, lay with the individual. To the younger generation that came to maturity in the 1870s and 1880s, on the other hand, the establishment of a conclusive relationship between specific disease entities and bacteriological organisms altered the relationship between patient and physician. Whereas Jarvis gave ultimate responsibility for health to the individual, his successors increasingly arrogated to themselves far greater authority over behavioral norms and health-related issues. The status and authority of the medical profession in the eyes of a new generation of physicians were derived from the possession of specialized knowledge and scientific training.

Having grown to maturity in a different milieu, Jarvis remained relatively untouched by the intellectual and scientific changes that were altering American medicine. There is no evidence that he was aware of medical developments in Germany and France; he remained faithful to the familiar code of his earlier years. The final fifteen years of his life were largely a reaffirmation of the underlying principles that had always given coherence to his life and career.

I

Although Jarvis had largely given up his psychiatric and medical practice by the mid-1860s, he continued to give frequent lectures on the laws of health and related topics, to say nothing about his contributions to the federal census of 1870.[2] Nor did his concern with the affairs of the Bay State diminish. In 1868 he was instrumental in persuading the legislature to launch an investigation into the abnormally high infant mortality rate at the state's almshouses.[3] The following year he became involved in a new drive to establish a state board of health. His abortive efforts years before had not dampened his enthusiasm. The report of the joint committee appointed by the legislature in the spring of 1869 undoubtedly met with his approval, for it urged the establishment of a state board of health and vital statistics "with such powers as will enable them thoroughly to investigate matters relating to public health, with a view to advise concerning it; but without any authoritative control or right of active interference."[4]

Although there was little direct opposition to the founding of a state board, it was clear that Jarvis's conception of the board's function and authority was not in accord with the views of some colleagues, notably Henry I. Bowditch and George Derby. In the memorial prepared for the Boston Sanitary Association in 1861, Jarvis had expressed the conviction that the basic function of such a board was to supervise the collection of vital statistics; he urged that it be given control of the state census and registration system. Bowditch and Derby held differing views. Both were firm believers in the efficacy of direct medical intervention; they wanted to link the authority of the state with the knowledge of the physician in order to manipulate those environmental conditions that determined health. Statistics in their eyes were important not because they revealed the operations of natural laws, but because they were instruments of change. Bowditch and Derby stood midway between the older voluntaristic tradition symbolized by Jarvis and an emerging tradition that shifted responsibility from the individual to an enlightened professional elite whose authority and status were derived from the possession of specialized knowledge.[5]

Given such differing conceptions, it was not surprising that friction would result. While the bill was still before the general court, Bowditch expressed regret that Jarvis had taken such a determined stand about "the *necessity* of Registration being *connected* with a Board of Health" and insisted that such a board could perform valuable functions without any involvement with registration procedures. "Why then fly in the face of the State officials and excite their determined opposition as you have really done by suggesting that idea?" he asked Jarvis. "I was in hopes that by trying to carry the *simple idea* of such a Board, we could get what we have both long wished for. Now I fear we are to be foiled again. I write plainly because I really think you hurt a cause we both have at heart by claiming too much at once. We are like beggars asking a *loaf* & refusing an ounce."[6]

In June 1869 the general court enacted and the governor signed the statute establishing a state board of health. Vague in its provisions, the law did not assign to the new agency responsibility for the registration of vital statistics. The absence of statutory powers of intervention in health-related matters, however, did not prove an impediment to the rapid expansion of the scope of the new board's authority; within a decade it had assumed a position of national leadership. Bowditch and Derby were among the seven appointees; they were elected chairman and secretary, respectively. Both men—but particularly Bowditch— were now prepared to use the board as the vehicle to protect the victims of preventable disease. The views of these two organizationally minded men prevailed, partly because of the apathy of the other five members. Nor did opposition from local authorities prove a deterrent; within a short period of time they had launched investigations of conditions in slaughter houses and tenement slums.[7]

While the board was being organized, Jarvis wrote to Bowditch and repeated his own views of its functions.[8] Despite his differences with Bowditch and Derby, Jarvis managed to persuade them to publish two long papers that summarized his life-long creed. His study of infant mortality appeared in 1872; his analysis of the political economy of health was published a year later. Both papers underscored the losses sustained by society through illness and premature death.[9]

Could government aid in improving the qualitative and quantitative aspects of human life? In his paper on the political economy of health Jarvis responded in the affirmative. Indeed, he was now prepared to concede to government broader responsibilities than he had at any time in the past. Perhaps the growth of a modernized society made him less sanguine about the future. Government, he insisted, had three basic powers: it could permit and forbid; it could grant privileges; and it could educate, advise, and encourage. When confronted with urban problems, for example, government could act positively to prevent the creation of unhealthy districts. "Every law, grant, or privilege from the legislature should have this invariable condition: that human health, strength or comfort should, in no manner or degree, be impaired or vitiated thereby." The welfare of the community, in other words, took precedence.[10]

Jarvis's acquiescence in the use of governmental authority was an expression of his own commitment to the idea of progress and the redemptive powers of education. At the very same time that he countenanced an expansion in state authority, he wrote two articles for the United States commissioner of education in which he reaffirmed his belief in the importance of education.[11] Beneath the surface, however, lurked a certain ambiguity. If the electorate was less than moral or enlightened (as the continued persistence of social problems seemed to indicate), how could government transcend such imperfections? Why would an imperfect electorate select morally superior officials? Often disparaging in his comments about the tone of American political life, Jarvis saw no inherent contradiction in asking public officials to rise above their constituents. He assumed that the American people, being rational, however imperfect, would recognize, trust, and follow leaders with superior education, moral fiber, and intelligence, thereby preventing any misuse of public authority.

II

By the third quarter of the nineteenth century new social problems had created greater receptivity toward structural innovation. The fascination with quantitative data had already given rise to a form of social research whose distinctiveness was its taxonomical character. Convinced that social science (to use the term that had come into vogue) made possible the control and manipulation of the environment, its supporters began to organize in order to enhance the possibility of applying soon-to-be-discovered laws to society. Influenced by the British National Association for the Promotion of Social Science (founded in 1857), a group of Bostonians that included the members of the Massachusetts Board of State Charities founded the American Social Science Association in 1865. Linking Baconian science with social activism, the association's basic objective was to develop "scientific" solutions to social problems "and to guide the public mind to the best practical means of promoting the Amendment of Laws, the Advancement of Education, the Prevention and Repression of Crime, the Reformation of Criminals, and the progress of Public Morality, the adoption of Sanitary Regulations, and the diffusion of sound principles on questions of Economy, Trade, and Finance." The confidence of the association's membership, on the other hand, was tempered in part by fear of unrestricted immigration and concern that the quality of American life was being eroded rapidly by corruption, selfishness, and venality. Composed of individuals drawn from the elite and the intelligentsia of the Northeast, the association sought no fundamental changes in American society; it wanted to make certain that the "best men" would retain a dominant position and thus prevent irresponsible elements from exercising undue power. The time had come for intelligent, moral, and educated men to take firm action to reverse the impending decline.[12]

Jarvis was among the founders of the new association and presided over its first meeting in October 1865. Here, after all, was still another vehicle for the dissemination of the principles of health and morality. Jarvis was immediately elected to the nominating committee and subsequently served on the executive committee and as one of the four members of the departmental committee on health. His hopes for the new organization, however, were never fully realized. Standing midway between an older generation reared with a commitment to moral philosophy and Baconian science and a newer one groping toward a modern concept of professionalization, the association never clearly defined its goals. In its early years its members were involved in public welfare, health, mortality, the census, sewerage disposal, civil service reform, free trade, sound currency, and honest politics.[13]

By 1869 the association had matured sufficiently to hold its first general meeting in New York City, where papers on a variety of subjects were presented. Among the participants was Friedrich Kapp, who read a paper that attempted to specify the relative contributions of immigration to the growth of the American population since 1790.[14] Working with figures taken from the seventh and eighth censuses, Kapp concluded that immigrants and their descendants accounted for twenty-one million out of a total population of about thirty million.[15]

Kapp's thesis was not novel; during the previous two decades there had been numerous warnings that aliens were threatening to overwhelm the old native stock and that American society was being disrupted by the dissolute and immoral behavior of such groups. By the 1880s and 1890s fear of aliens would help to create a mature racial ideology among (but not limited to) New England Brahmins and a movement to end unrestricted immigration. During the early 1870s, however, the elements of fear and anxiety that would become so pronounced in the future remained submerged. The census of 1870 was a portent of things to come, for Francis A. Walker specifically went out of his way to warn that the fertility of the native population was declining rapidly. This decline, he noted in ominous terms, was ''covered from the common sight by a flood of immigration unprecedented in history.'' The public, he added, ''still fails to apprehend the full significance of the decline in the rate of national increase.'' Although it would be nearly two decades before Walker's hostility toward aliens would fully surface, his portrayal of immigrants in unflattering terms was already evident.[16]

Kapp's essay immediately aroused Jarvis's concern. Since he had criticized Jesse Chickering and Joseph C.G. Kennedy for comparable estimates nearly two decades earlier, it was understandable that he would subject Kapp's analysis to equally careful scrutiny.[17] Often portraying the Irish in unflattering terms,

Jarvis never abandoned his basic environmentalism and belief in the possibility of assimilation. His faith in the rationality and lawfulness of the universe always acted as a counterforce to the more pessimistic interpretation that explained the origins of social problems in harsh hereditarian terms. Consequently, he was hostile to Kapp's paper for two reasons: it rested on erroneous data and a false methodology, and it also implied the genetic inferiority of certain groups.

In 1870 Jarvis concluded that the matter could not be permitted to rest; he decided to prepare an article for the *Atlantic Monthly* rebutting the claim that immigrants were rapidly overwhelming the native population. The paper was finally published in the spring of 1872 after being read before a meeting of the American Academy of Arts and Sciences. The article began with a summary of the views of statisticians, particularly Louis Schade[18] and Kapp, who believed that fertility rates of older groups had fallen markedly in America. "In harmony with these views," Jarvis observed, "are some seemingly wild opinions as to the number of people of foreign births living now in the United States." To deal with these exaggerated opinions he proposed to determine the approximate number of foreigners and their descendants in the United States between 1800 and 1870. The bulk of the article was devoted to a careful evaluation of existing data sources, particularly the census. Besides repeating earlier criticisms of the census, he noted that the statistics purporting to show the excess of births over deaths were totally erroneous.[19]

"There is not only no ground for the theory of the limited growth of the American, and of the unlimited growth of the foreign, element in the population of the United States," Jarvis informed his readers, "but, on the contrary, the natural increase is at a lower rate in the foreign than in the American families." Reworking the available data with new assumptions based on life expectancy, age distribution, and various mortality and other statistical records, he came up with an entirely different conclusion. Jarvis estimated that the foreign-born and their descendants who came to the United States after 1790 numbered between 10,500,000 and 11,600,000, and perhaps fewer. Though drawing no conclusions beyond his rejection of the estimates of Schade and Kapp, the thrust of his remarks was unmistakably clear. He seemed to unequivocally reject a nascent but growing fear that the native-born stock (those who had come before 1790) faced progressive extinction.[20]

There remained, nevertheless, an underlying element of ambiguity in Jarvis's mind about the future. His universalistic view inhibited a turn in the direction of those Brahmins who were steadily moving toward an ideology that made race the crucial determinant of culture. Yet Jarvis did not remain unaffected by the new currents around him. At a conference in 1873 sponsored jointly by the American Social Science Association and the newly founded American Public Health Association, Jarvis spoke extemporaneously on the vital statistics of different races to an audience composed of members of state and city boards of health. "There is much in race," he conceded at the outset. "The races differ more than we imagine." Vitality was not equally distributed, and there were differences in the proportion of births to marriages and in life expectancy. The Irish in particular had the highest mortality rate among their young (as compared with the experiences of fourteen other nations). In the United States generally foreigners during the first seven decades of the nineteenth century had far higher death rates than natives; for every 100 deaths among the latter there were 179 among the former. "Somehow or other, I do not know how it is," mused Jarvis with obvious puzzlement, "but the old families are the most enduring, most persistent, and have the longest life."[21]

Perhaps confidence in the native population inhibited the development of harsher feelings. Nevertheless, the fact that Jarvis employed a racial typology was not without some significance, even if his definition of race was obscure. By 1875 his concern had become even more pronounced. In a letter to Walker he compared the brief working life of Irish Celts with the longer ones of Scandinavians, Germans, and Anglo-Saxons, a fact that political economists could not afford to ignore. "Tis true," he wrote in an uncharacteristic tone, "we cannot discriminate & exclude the weak liver & admit only the strong & enduring. But we cannot rejoice over the arrival of those who bring low vitality as we should over those richly endowed with life." The greatest contribution to the United States came from Teutonic, Scandinavian, and Anglo-Saxons groups; all others had a lower vital force. When intermarriage came in the future—as it surely would—"it will be at the cost of the better life, the weak will contribute their lower vitality & the result will be a depreciation of the children below the strength of the Saxon parents. And thus, as far as this goes the average vitality of the American people will fall to the average of the weak & the stronger elements."[22]

Any organized effort to bring together individuals who shared a common commitment to problems related to health and environment was to be encouraged. When the American Public Health Association was founded in 1872, Jarvis immediately gave the new organization his hearty approval. Conceding that there was always the danger that individuals with more "imagination than knowledge, [and] more zeal than wisdom" might be enlisted, he nevertheless felt that the movement represented by the new association was "one of the essential elements in the advance of civilization & one of the necessities of the age."[23] Like the American Social Science Association, the American Public Health Association brought together physicians, sanitary engineers, and public-spirited citizens, all of whom shared a commitment to social uplift. In its early days the association had not yet moved in the direction of justifying its authority by reference to the possession of expertise that could only be transmitted through formal training and certified by peer review. Consequently, its program was extraordinarily broad; most of its members were determined to alleviate any and all conditions that inhibited health and promoted disease.[24]

The fact that many of the founding members of the American Public Health Association exemplified a happy combination of character, morality, and knowledge only stimulated Jarvis's enthusiasm. As a figure who had been associated with sanitary science for more than a quarter of a century, he was immediately called upon to take an active role. His absence from the preliminary organizing sessions did not prevent his election to membership and appointment to the executive committee. Indeed, Dr. Elisha Harris asked him, as "the master in this field," to give a report on vital and anthropological statistics. For some unknown reason, Jarvis did not comply with this request. Instead he prepared a paper for the spring meeting of the association in 1873 on the relationship between war and famine on the one hand and marriages and births on the other. Six months later he delivered another report on the role and responsibility of women for the health of their families. That the new association saw fit to listen to such papers was testimony to its basic character. Responsibility for health could not be left in the hands of scientists and physicians alone; its maintenance required the active participation of all.[25]

III

During his twilight years Jarvis continued to be active in psychiatry. On occasion he appeared as an expert witness in court. With the single exception of the Webster trial, few of these proceedings were controversial. Toward the end of 1868, however, he became involved in the state's most prominent murder trial since the Webster case nearly two decades earlier. The facts of the case were simple. Samuel M. Andrews, an individual who had led an exemplary life, murdered Cornelius Holmes, a friend who had made Andrews his heir. Andrews testified that on several occasions Holmes had attempted to commit sodomy on his person. On the evening of the murder Holmes threw Andrews down and again attempted to have homosexual relations. Andrews then struck Holmes with several stones and then claimed to have lost all consciousness of subsequent acts. A post-mortem examination indicated that Holmes had received more than twenty blows with stones that weighed up to four pounds each.[26]

During the trial the prosecution maintained that Andrews committed murder in order to inherit the bulk of the estate. An effort to prove robbery failed, for the victim was found with a large sum of money on his body. Counsel for the defense attempted to prove that the defendant was insane at the time of the crime, and retained Jarvis as an expert witness. In his testimony Jarvis argued that Andrews suffered from *mania transitoria*, a form of mental disorder that appeared suddenly in persons previously sound, had a brief duration, and just as quickly disappeared. During his testimony the judge ruled that Jarvis could not refer to other psychiatric authorities. In his charge to the jury he told the members that the "opinions of experts are mere evidence for the jury to consider" and then remarked that "the opinions of experts are not so highly regarded now as they formerly were, for while they often afford great aid in determining facts, it often happens that experts can be found to testify to any theory, however absurd." The prosecution in turn called Dr. George H. Choate, superintendent of the Taunton State Lunatic Hospital. Choate testified that the existence of insanity in a given family was no proof that any individual member was so afflicted; he also denied that *mania transitoria* was a disease.[27]

In his summation the prosecutor relied upon the M'Naghten precedent. An individual could be absolved of criminal responsibility, he told the jury, only when "incapable of appreciating the difference between right and wrong . . . or when, by reason of disease, his will is overborne, so that he can no longer exercise control over his actions." Passion and violence were not to be equated with insanity. The prosecutor also attempted to discredit Jarvis, who conceded that he had never encountered an actual case of *mania transitoria.* To accept Jarvis's testimony would ultimately lead to the destruction of the criminal law by surrendering its administration to physicians. In his charge to the jury the judge listed four possible options. If the defendant acted in self-defense, he was to be acquitted; if, under the provocation of an assault, he exceeded the proper limits of self-defense, he could be convicted of manslaughter; he could also be found guilty as charged or not guilty by reason of insanity. Ultimately the jury found Andrews guilty of manslaughter, for which he was sentenced to twenty years in prison.[28]

Jarvis's reaction to the trial and its outcome was one of anger. He was especially critical of the presiding judge, noting with contempt his hostile attitude toward psychiatric testimony. Not content to let matters rest, he immediately prepared two long articles, which were published in both the *American Journal of Insanity* and the *Boston Medical and Surgical Journal.* The first summarized the views of European and American authorities who accepted the reality of *mania transitoria.* The characteristics of this form of insanity, Jarvis insisted, were clear: mania could appear suddenly and without warning; it could manifest itself in a single act of violence; the act could go beyond its original purpose; the mania could cease and leave no trace; during the paroxysms the individual could be unconscious of the act; and after the return of sanity there might be no conscious feeling of guilt. The second article was a critical account of the trial, particularly of the verdict. The members of the jury, noted Jarvis, accepted Andrews' veracity when it convicted him of manslaughter; otherwise they would have found him guilty of murder. Yet they rejected the defendant's claim that he had no memory of the episode.[29]

The positions taken by both sides during the trial reflected the ambivalent attitudes of many Americans in the late nineteenth century. Given social and economic change, how could citizens maintain traditional values if institutional dislocations undermined the moral consensus? The conflict between law and psychiatry evolved around this very question. A decade after the Andrews case the controversy would gain national prominence when Charles J. Guiteau was tried for the murder of President James A. Garfield. Interestingly enough, Jarvis's argument rested on a hereditarian foundation; he interpreted Andrews' act as a manifestation of an inherited disease. The difficulty that he faced was that an environmental explanation of Andrews' action would have surely led to a verdict of guilty as charged; evil was the result of free choices made by human beings. In this respect Jarvis was not atypical; in the Guiteau case the psychiatrists testifying for the defense also employed hereditarian reasoning in arguing for a verdict of not guilty by reason of insanity. The prosecution in the Andrews case, however, specifically rejected the allegation that insanity was an inherited malady. Evil was the result of volitional action; it was far easier to conceal a criminal intent than an insane mind. Above all, the prosecutor explicitly warned that if Jarvis's latitudinarian claims were accepted, the "social interests of society" would be ignored. The very same point was echoed in an article in the Boston *Transcript*. A broad interpretation of insanity, in other words, would further contribute toward the subversion of the social and moral order; those who were concerned with the maintenance of stability and morality simply could not accept the views represented by Jarvis.[30]

Such contrasting positions cannot be interpreted solely in terms of a simple dichotomy between law and psychiatry; within the ranks of the latter specialty Jarvis's position was equally controversial. At the meetings of the Association of Medical Superintendents of American Institutions for the Insane two years later a debate occurred over Jarvis's paper. John P. Gray, the authoritarian editor of the *American Journal of Insanity* who would later become one of the star witnesses for the government in the Guiteau trial, used the occasion to attack Jarvis when another member alluded to *mania transitoria* as an established disease entity. Although Gray would argue during the Guiteau trial that there was a fundamental distinction between character demoralization and evil on the one hand and insanity on the other, his disagreements with Jarvis were not yet phrased in such terms. Gray simply insisted that *mania transitoria* was too vague a category; it had no definite symptoms "by which we are to characterize such a form and separate it from a general class." The ensuing discussion was revealing, for the issue of moral insanity (perhaps the most controversial concept in nineteenth-century psychiatry) was immediately introduced into the discussion. Moral insanity (defined as a disease that affected primarily the emotions and not the thought process or the intellect) was the pivotal point about which the entire problem of the relationship between crime, society, and evil revolved. To accept such a concept seemed extraordinarily dangerous to some. It implied the absence of any innate moral faculty, which in turn raised the possibility of a thoroughgoing materialism and perhaps the very denial of the idea that human beings were responsible for their behavior. Unfortunately Jarvis did not attend the meeting, and there is no way of determining the position that he might have taken. Certainly his colleagues were unable to come to any firm decision; there was a distinct effort to escape from the ramifications that flowed from a full acceptance of moral insanity.[31]

At about this time Jarvis's dissatisfaction with traditional institutional care crystallized. His experiences with patients in his home and observations of British practices had convinced him that other approaches might be more effective. In this respect he was not alone, for interest in decentralized hospitals modeled along the lines of the colony system in Gheel, Belgium, was on the rise. Within Massachusetts a controversy raged over the recommendation by the superintendent of the Worcester State Lunatic Hospital that the state build a new physical plant according to a decentralized plan; in several other states the situation was much the same. The conflict threatened to split institutional psychiatrists into warring factions.[32]

In 1870 Jarvis leaped into the fray by circulating a paper on the care of the insane that seemed to break with the cherished tenets of the Association of Medical Superintendents of American Institutions for the Insane. Indeed, John Curwen, a friend and superintendent of the Pennsylvania State Lunatic Hospital, urged Jarvis not to carry out his intention to publish the paper in the *Atlantic,* for this would necessitate a public reply to its unorthodoxy. The discussion, implied Curwen, more properly belonged within the association. Jarvis went along with Curwen's suggestion, although he did arrange to have the paper published in early 1872 in the annual report of the Massachusetts State Board of Health for 1871.[33]

The first part of Jarvis's paper was relatively uncontroversial; it repeated most of the generalizations accepted by the overwhelming majority of his colleagues. But then he posed a seemingly innocuous question. Given the varied nature of insanity, were traditional congregate hospitals "adapted to the various conditions and wants of all classes of patients"? His negative response came as a shock to many of his fellow delegates who had labored unceasingly to codify the principles that made the congregate hospital virtually the only legitimate form. In its early days, conceded Jarvis, the traditional hospital served an indispensable function. But it was no longer appropriate for a different age. Originally the congregate hospital was intended to care for "a dangerous element of humanity"; hence it took a characteristic architectural form. Most public hospitals had a large central building with wings extending on both sides. Such a plan facilitated careful supervision; strong doors and barred windows reinforced security. However, continued Jarvis, hospitals ought to be arranged "to meet the varied wants, capacities and liabilities of the inmates.'' An institution devoted to custody did little to enhance the self-respect of inmates, which was a vital ingredient in any successful therapy. Many patients did not require confinement. What was needed was a variety of structures, each serving the need of particular groups. Such a hospital system would also overcome community distrust; congregate institutions designed with security as the overriding consideration simply reinforced public fears that mentally ill persons constituted a real menace to the community.[34]

The issues raised by Jarvis were of a particularly sensitive nature. During the preceding decade mental hospitals and superintendents had come under attack by critics who charged that commitment procedures often deprived mentally ill persons of their civil rights. The exposés by former patients—notably those of Mrs. E.P.W. Packard—added fuel to the controversy. When a number of state legislatures conducted investigations of institutional practices and debated the merits of personal liberty statutes designed to protect insane patients and limit involuntary commitment, superintendents were thrown on the defensive. Although Jarvis did not share the beliefs of critics of psychiatry, his colleagues were disturbed by the implications of his recommendations.[35]

At the meetings of the association in June 1871 Jarvis's paper was the subject of a lengthy discussion. From the outset it was clear that there was strong opposition to his views. The opening comments by his old friend Isaac Ray—which were seconded by Thomas S. Kirkbride and John P. Gray—were indicative of the prevailing sentiment. Ray defended existing architectural arrangements, which facilitated effective medical supervision and were more economical and efficient. The declining character of the attendant corps, furthermore, made maintenance of the status quo indispensable. A decentralized system was also incompatible with adequate security considerations. Others seconded Ray's comments. Gray went so far as to insist that "opinions of men without practical experience should not have great weight," an obvious allusion to the fact that Jarvis had never served as a hospital superintendent. From the tone of the debate it was evident that Jarvis had few supporters.[36]

Having entered psychiatry at a time when the overwhelming

majority of the insane were confined in welfare and penal institutions, the majority of association members were not inclined to change direction. In their eyes, responsibility for existing failures was attributable to the refusal of American society to meet its obligations toward the mentally ill. Decentralized institutions and boarding-out plans seemed to threaten their autonomy and integrity, for both impinged upon the central role of the superintendent as stipulated by the principles of moral treatment. More importantly, they believed that decentralization meant additional overcrowding, the isolation of the chronic insane, and an end to therapeutic goals, all of which implied a rejection of therapeutic care. Consequently, they resisted what they regarded as illegitimate and dangerous attacks on themselves or their institutions. When the plan to build a new decentralized state hospital in Worcester was defeated (a plan that Jarvis endorsed), Ray, Kirkbride, and Earle all breathed a sigh of relief at the outcome.[37]

Jarvis had spent his career in an entirely different social setting; he was far more receptive to a pluralistic system. As a partial outsider, he lacked any commitment to a particular structural form. Recognizing a kindred soul, a European psychiatrist who migrated to the United States wrote to Jarvis and expressed the opinion that lack of *"individual treatment"* was the *"common defect."* Offering no treatment, he concluded, violated the rights of patients when they were placed in institutions without therapeutic facilities.[38] Jarvis's age and lack of institutional leverage, however, rendered him powerless to serve as a mediating force. While his colleagues endorsed his endeavors to promote the collection of uniform hospital statistics, they were not in the slightest disposed toward modifying their commitment to congregate institutions. Jarvis's plea, therefore, fell on deaf ears.[39]

IV

As Jarvis entered the eighth decade of life, his thoughts slowly turned toward the past. In 1873 he completed an autobiography that ran to no less than 327 handwritten pages.[40] Generally accurate, it conveyed a sense of pride and achievement; gone were the doubts and fears that had been present in his younger years. Although self-criticism was by no means absent, its tone was one of confidence in the future. Nor had Jarvis's faith in God and the moral character of the universe in any way diminished; he remained committed to the Unitarian creed that had served as an anchor since his early years. If anything, his career as a physician only confirmed his faith that divine law gave medicine its raison d'être. In this sense he was far removed from European medicine and its emphasis on clinical observation and laboratory research. A world separated his generation from the new generation of young Americans who went abroad in ever-growing numbers in the 1870s and thereafter to study medicine. To Jarvis the function of the physician was not cure but prevention, and preventive medicine could not be separated from the moral order of the universe.[41]

In early 1874 Jarvis suffered a stroke, which left him partially paralyzed. For the first time in his life he had to curtail his activities sharply. Although requests for the presentation of papers and the preparation of articles continued to arrive with regularity, he was forced to decline or defer all of them because of his physical condition. News of his illness brought forth expressions of sympathy and concern from many colleagues. Fortunately, Almira was able to care for her incapacitated husband and assist him with his extensive correspondence. Within the limitations mandated by his illness, Jarvis continued to work when able.[42]

For many years Jarvis had retained an unflagging interest in his family genealogy, but his researches were too incomplete to be put into finished form. As the years advanced, more and more his thoughts turned to his beloved Concord, whose origin and subsequent development seemed to parallel his own life. Over the years he had accumulated a considerable body of material pertaining to its history and genealogy. Now, confined to his house, he began to prepare a study of Concord that was at the same time autobiographical in nature.[43]

In spite of ill health and failing eyesight, Jarvis completed in 1880 a manuscript of over six hundred pages dealing with the social and domestic history of Concord during the century ending in 1878. A labor of love, the work reflected Jarvis's admiration for and attachment to his place of birth and his unyielding conviction that development and progress were synonymous. Unlike other romantic critics who saw American history in terms of decline, he saw it in terms of upward movement toward a more ideal social order. The work itself brought together an impressive collection of details, many of which were drawn from his own memories of his youth. Throughout the tone was one of unrelieved celebration.[44]

Jarvis's love affair with Concord, however, was not yet finished, for he immediately undertook to re-create Concord as it had existed between 1810 and 1820. Besides locating every physical structure, he compiled biographical sketches of most of the town's residents. Aside from the intrinsic value of the work (completed in manuscript form in 1883), he found extraordinary satisfaction in returning to his childhood and youth "to revive and revel in the scenes and impressions" that had become his "absorbing happiness." At the age of eighty Jarvis enveloped Concord in a glowing mantle. His earlier failure in that community left no residual bitterness; his subsequent success wiped out whatever frustration or unhappiness remained.[45]

In studying Concord, Jarvis also turned to a question that was beginning to trouble older families whose ancestors had migrated to Massachusetts in the seventeenth century. Jarvis remained oblivious to the claim that the superiority of America's native population was being threatened by hordes of immigrants. His analysis (parts of which were published) showed a fundamentally different pattern. Comparing those individuals and families who resided in Concord between 1635 and 1700 with the voting list of 1881, he noted that a large proportion of the first group had indeed disappeared. His explanation, however, was largely in nonpejorative terms. The remoteness of Concord and the absence of economic opportunities for many encouraged outmigration. Hence the families that had left Concord had not disappeared but were "as full and as strong as ever, with a fair prospect of being followed by a line of posterity in perpetual succession of generations" elsewhere in the state and nation.[46]

Aside from research on the history of Concord, the final decade of Jarvis's life was uneventful. Unable to travel because of illness, he slowly resigned from all of the medical and scholarly organizations to which he belonged, including the American Academy of Arts and Sciences and the Norfolk District Medical Society. In 1883 he finally gave up the presidency of the American Statistical Association after thirty-one years in office. His fellow members promptly elected him president-emeritus and adopted a warm and touching resolution "calling attention to the high rank which he has gained as a writer on statistical and physiological subjects, and to the benefits which he has conferred upon his fellow men by his laborious investigations, particularly in vital statistics, which have made him an honor to his country and to science."[47]

During the late 1870s, Jarvis's health deteriorated still furthur. In 1880 he broke his hip after being thrown from a carriage while on a visit to Concord and was confined to bed for the better part of a year. The illness of his wife necessitated the employment of a full-time housekeeper. Fortunately, the couple's financial resources were more than adequate for the exigencies of old age. Fastidious to the end, Jarvis made meticulous provision for the disposition of his valuable library, which was given to the American Statistical Association. Aside from some modest bequests to his housekeeper and to Harvard College, the bulk of the estate was left to nieces and nephews on both sides of the family. On October 17, 1884, Jarvis felt well enough to attend a meeting of the American Statistical Association for the first time in a year. Three days later he suffered another stroke and died on October 31. Almira, who had been confined to bed by illness and the infirmities of age, revived sufficiently to settle all of the details of her husband's funeral. As though her life was also completed, she passed away two days later. On November 5 a joint funeral service was held for Almira and Edward Jarvis in the Dorchester church which they had faithfully attended for four decades. Immediately thereafter they were buried in Sleepy Hollow Cemetery in their beloved Concord. United in marriage for half a century, they remained together in death as well.[48]

"For more than fifty years," an acquaintance wrote in a touching tribute, "they had lived together in mutual love and helpfulness. Their lives had come to be assimilated in spirit, tone, and habit, so that the virtues and tasks of each were reflected in the other. Each seemed to be necessary to the other, and their lives were so beautifully interwoven that those who knew them could only think with pain of one being taken and the other left. But these who had made the journey of life together were not to be separated when they came to the river. . . . Like Saul and Jonathan, 'lovely and pleasant were they in their lives, and in death they were not divided.' ''[49]

Jarvis's last article, which was published posthumously in a leading Unitarian periodical, remained true to the religious faith and moral code that gave coherence and meaning to his life. Emphasizing the relationship between proper nutrition and health, he expressed regret over the widespread ignorance of the "Law of Life." His final words portrayed his lifelong concerns: "We therefore need a more general education in the law of life, in the principles of health, and in regard to the means by which strength is created and vigor maintained." No better epitaph could have summed up his career.[50]

V

Shortly after his death Jarvis was the subject of several memoirs prepared by close friends. Andrew P. Peabody, whom he had known since college days and who subsequently edited the *North American Review* and taught at Harvard, published a moving piece in the *New England Historical and Genealogical Register*. Robert W. Wood, another long-standing friend active in the American Statistical Association, delivered an address at a meeting of that organization in January 1885, and a member of the Concord Social Circle wrote a lengthy biographical article. Appreciative obituaries also appeared in the *Boston Medical and Surgical Journal* and the proceedings of the American Antiquarian Society and the American Academy of Arts and Sciences. Written by different authors, all of these notices emphasized a common theme—namely, the inseparable relationship between science and statistics on the one hand and religion and morality on the other. The purpose to which Jarvis consecrated himself, noted Wood, was "the intellectual and moral uplifting and the amelioration of the physical condition of man," a judgment echoed by the other eulogies. Science was more than simply the objectification of the world; without a moral dimension scientific laws were meaningless. Whether or not they were aware of it, all of the eulogists were describing not only Jarvis's career but also the character of medicine in the mid-nineteenth century.[51]

Edward Jarvis typified, as much as an individual can, an approach that briefly altered the basic character of American medicine. Reared in a devout household, instructed in Unitarian theology, trained in Common Sense philosophy, committed to a Baconian interpretation of science, and influenced by the rising doubt about the efficacy of traditional therapeutics, Jarvis contributed to a newer synthesis that merged medicine, morality, and social activism. Just as his understanding of pathology was expressed in moral terms, so he defined the role of physician in comparable terms. Andrew P. Peabody, whose own ministerial and academic career paralleled that of his friend, grasped this vital fact when he described the breadth of Jarvis's writings, which included "the treatment of the insane, sanitary laws and measures, physical, mental and moral education, and the causes and remedies of vice and crime." Jarvis, added Peabody in perceptive terms, "never wrote except with philanthropic purpose; and on many subjects now of general interest, his were pioneer essays, designed and adapted to wake the public mind to pressing needs and urgent claims." What this implied, of course, was that science led unerringly to philanthropy, a term that in the nineteenth century included an extraordinarily wide range of activities that cut across the public and private sectors. To figures of Jarvis's mold, the profession of medicine derived its legitimacy from its philanthropic efforts; physicians, by discovering operative natural laws, provided humanity with the understanding that was so vital to the proper conduct of life. Therapeutic intervention in cases of disease, on the other hand, was ineffective because traditional remedies rarely served their intended purpose and, more importantly, did not touch the conditions that gave rise to disease. For this very reason medicine was defined in taxonomical terms; proper classification systems and appropriate statistical data were the true bases for continued progress. Like other contemporary figures, Jarvis had few doubts

about the possibilities of progress; he shared the almost un-
bounded optimism and hope for a better world characteristic of
his generation.[52]

Admittedly, Jarvis's analysis of the social and medical problems facing his countrymen was often from the perspective of
one who had never experienced firsthand the lives of those most
touched by the consequences of urbanization and industrialization. Nor did he consider that the supposed beneficiaries of
moral and medical uplift were more victims than agents of evil
and immorality. But he never imposed, at least in modern
terms, a purely hereditarian explanation for social failures. At
heart he assumed that all human beings possessed freedom and
rationality, thereby providing them with the potential for
meaningful change. The role of medicine—a role that defined
its intrinsic function—was to discover and to specify those conditions that promoted health and reduced morbidity and mortality. Once this was accomplished, the thrust to eliminate pressing
social and individual evils would become all but irresistible.
Given rationality (and even self-interest), men everywhere
would freely comply with divine moral imperatives, thereby rendering superfluous the use of government authority. Jarvis's
commitment to a voluntaristic political ideology was a natural
concomitant of his larger view of society and the universe.

Jarvis's importance lay precisely in his efforts to unify medicine, science, and religion. Unlike some of his European contemporaries whose contributions to pathology were increasingly
derived from a laboratory and clinical setting, Jarvis's habitat
was all of society. Disease could not be understood apart from
individual behavior or the state of society. Nor was the presumed order of the physical world merely imposed by the
human mind; the orderliness of the universe was a reality that
could be described in statistical terms. To a nation experiencing
rapid social change and yet committed to certain religious
tenets, the careers of men like Jarvis had considerable appeal.
For Jarvis offered both an explanation of the present and hope
for the future within an intellectual framework that buttressed
rather than denied dominant religious and moral assumptions.
Consequently, he and others like him were accorded recognition
and status by an appreciative community.

By the time of his death, however, Jarvis and the views he represented had been relegated to an irrelevant past by a new generation of physicians and scientists who were rapidly altering the structure of the medical profession and redefining its basic concepts. The specific germ theory of disease represented the newer trends. The proper place for the physician became the research laboratory. Broad environmental issues were of concern only insofar as they influenced the specific organisms that caused disease; religion represented an entirely separate sphere. The physician now became a scientist rather than an educator or philanthropist; the authority of medicine was justified by its possession of forms of knowledge and expertise available only to a select few. In this new world, which was dominated by a bewildering number of professional organizations and specialties, Jarvis was an alien. His view of the function of the physician seemed the vestigial remnant of a bygone age, and his social approach to the prevention of disease was overwhelmed by a molecularly oriented conception of disease. Even when his successors spoke about prevention, their model was not an environmental one; prevention in their eyes was a function of some artificially induced immunity. Moreover, for the bulk of practitioners the focus continued to remain on the individual patient; social medicine was always honored more in theory than in practice. Even those who pursued a medical career within public health often restricted the scope of their activities; by the early twentieth century public health was dominated less by broad social and environmental concerns and more by the thrust to identify specific disease organisms and the discovery and production of appropriate antitoxins or means of immunization.

Yet Jarvis's contributions would not be without considerable influence. Paradoxically, his work would have its greatest impact not upon medicine, but upon the emerging social and behavioral sciences, which by the late nineteenth century were beginning to assume their modern form. These sciences would define themselves in taxonomical terms; they would develop classification systems and rely upon the collection of statistical data to formulate broad generalizations capable of being applied to social problems. To a large degree their foundation was constructed by medical figures like Edward Jarvis. His *Report on In-*

sanity not only was the first major statistical survey of its kind, but also was a prototype of later social investigations. Similarly, his effort to modernize the census and to ensure that accurate and comparable statistical data would be available helped to create a body of materials that in the twentieth century would become the basis of most social and economic research and would also play an increasingly important role in policy formulation. Less tangible, although equally significant, was the part that he played in creating an awareness of the importance of morbidity and mortality patterns and the degree to which these patterns were related to the social and physical environment. Indeed, his emphasis on the necessity for a modernized census rested precisely upon his conviction that mortality patterns were the measure by which a society could be judged. During his lifetime and after his death this belief slowly but surely became a cardinal principle in a variety of disciplines even though his contributions were largely overlooked.

All of this is not to argue that Edward Jarvis was a modern social scientist. Unlike Jarvis, the latter emulated the language of the hard sciences and by so doing staked out claims for authority derived from the possession of specialized knowledge. Yet these very same individuals would largely ignore the ethical and moral issues that remained central to Jarvis's vision. For in his eyes activism was a means to an end that could be grasped only by a knowledge and understanding of the moral imperatives that grew out of broad religious truths.

It is of course true that few present-day scientists, physicians, or social scientists would accept Jarvis's religious faith, his voluntaristic philosophy that left with the individual ultimate responsibility for the maintenance of health, or his conviction that the orderly nature of the physical world was a reality created by a Divine Authority. On the other hand, the questions raised by Jarvis remain as compelling today as they were during his lifetime. Can scientific inquiry ever be separated from a moral dimension that deals with ends as well as means? Is it possible to define health and disease apart from an ethical system that embodies more than a statistical statement of normality? By what standards do human beings measure and judge environmentally related issues and problems? And how can the competing claims of individual freedom and public control be resolved without sacrificing one to maximize the other? These and other concerns were central to Jarvis's life. Perhaps the answers that he gave were neither appropriate nor applicable, but surely the questions remain as valid today as they were more than a century ago. In this sense the career of Edward Jarvis remains relevant to the concerns of the present.

Notes

ABBREVIATIONS

AAS American Antiquarian Society
ASA American Statistical Association
CFPL Concord Free Public Library
CLMHMS Countway Library of Medicine, Harvard Medical School
EJ Edward Jarvis
EJEL Edward Jarvis, European Letters
EJLB Edward Jarvis, Letter Books
HLHU Houghton Library, Harvard University
IPH Institute of the Pennsylvania Hospital
LC Library of Congress

INTRODUCTION

1. I am greatly indebted to Professor Barbara G. Rosenkrantz for permitting me to use her unpublished paper "The Search for Professional Order in 19th Century American Medicine," which was delivered at the Fourteenth International Congress of the History of Science, Tokyo, Japan, 1974.

CHAPTER 1

1. Lewis Mumford, *The Conduct of Life* (New York, 1951), 186; Timothy Dwight, *Travels in New England and New York,* ed. Barbara M. Solomon (4 vols.: Cambridge, 1969), I, 280–81. See also

Ralph Waldo Emerson, *A Historical Discourse Delivered before the Citizens of Concord, 12th September, 1835 on the Second Centennial Anniversary of the Incorporation of the Town* (Concord, 1835).

2. George Jarvis et al., *The Jarvis Family* (Hartford, 1879), 1–18, 234ff.; Benjamin H. Branch, Jr., *The Branch, Harris, Jarvis, and Chinn Book: A Family Outline* (Ann Arbor, 1964), 202ff.; *Concord, Massachusetts: Births, Marriages, and Deaths, 1635–1850* (Boston, 1895), passim. The latter source erroneously gives Edward Jarvis's birth as January 10. Originally he was named Asa; in 1821 his name was changed to Edward Asa Jarvis, and shortly thereafter he dropped the use of his middle name completely.

3. EJ, "Memoir of Francis Jarvis," in *Memoirs of Members of the Social Circle in Concord: Second Series from 1795 to 1840* (Cambridge, 1888), 30–51. This memoir was written in 1854.

4. This portrait of Francis Jarvis is drawn from EJ, "Diary" (2 mss. vols., 1827–1842), I, 95–96, CFPL; EJ, "Memoir of Francis Jarvis," 39–43, 46–48; EJ, "Traditions and Reminiscences of Concord Massachusetts, or a Contribution to the Social and Domestic History of the Town 1779 to 1878," 379–81, mss. vol., CFPL.

5. EJ, "Diary," I, 100, CFPL. For an equally unflattering description of Edward's oldest brother see Edward M. Emerson, "Memoir of Francis Jarvis, Jr.," in *Memoirs of Members of the Social Circle in Concord: Second Series,* 370–76. Emerson noted that Francis Jarvis, Jr., lacked "ambition, imagination, enthusiasm." He was disinterested in his father's bakery business and was glad to inherit the family farm, which provided him with a good living with minimal effort. He was particularly attracted by small details and spent considerable time in collecting statistics on various subjects.

6. This description of Concord is based upon EJ, "Traditions and Reminiscences," chap. 1 et passim, CFPL; EJ, "Houses & People. Concord Mass. 1810–1820," mss. vol., CFPL; and Lemuel Shattuck, *A History of the Town of Concord* (Boston, 1835). See also Robert A. Gross, *The Minutemen and Their World* (New York, 1976).

7. EJ, "Diary," I, 7, CFPL; EJ, "Traditions and Reminiscences," 301–8, CFPL.

8. Ezra Ripley, *The Obligation of Parents to Give their Children a Virtuous Education . . . Illustrated and Urged in a Sermon, Delivered, September 7, 1820* (Cambridge, 1820), 9–10. See also Ripley's *Half Century Discourse, Delivered November 16, 1828, at Concord, Massachusetts* (Concord, 1829) (copy originally owned by EJ and now in Boston Public Library), and Barzillai Frost and Convers Francis, *Two*

Sermons on the Death of Rev. Ezra Ripley, D.D. (Boston, 1841), and Ralph Waldo Emerson, "Memoir of Rev. Ezra Ripley, D.D.," in *The Centennial of the Social Circle in Concord March 21, 1882* (Cambridge, 1882), 168-76.

9. EJ, "Diary," I, 216, CFPL. See also EJ, "Autobiography," 327, mss. vol., HLHU; EJ, "Houses & People. Concord Mass. 1810-1820," 190-209, CFPL; and Jarvis's recollections of Ezra Ripley and Rev. Hersey B. Goodwin, January 25, 1881, typescript copy, CFPL. For a general summary of the relationship between religion and antebellum reform see John L. Thomas, "Romantic Reform in America, 1815-1865," *American Quarterly*, XVII (Winter 1965), 656-81, and the introduction by William G. McLoughlin to Charles G. Finney's *Lectures on Revivals of Religion* (Cambridge, 1960), vii-lii.

10. EJ, "Diary," I, 8-13, CFPL; EJ, "Autobiography," 2-3, HLHU.

11. EJ, "Diary," I, 14-31, CFPL; EJ, "Autobiography," 3-5, HLHU.

12. This discussion of moral philosophy at Harvard is based largely on Daniel Walker Howe, *The Unitarian Conscience: Harvard Moral Philosophy, 1805-1861* (Cambridge, 1970), passim. See also Samuel Eliot Morison, *Three Centuries of Harvard 1636-1936* (Cambridge, 1936), 195-245.

13. EJ, "Diary," I, 33-39, CFPL.

14. *A Catalogue of the Officers and Students of the University in Cambridge. October, 1825* (Cambridge, 1825), 21; A. Hunter Dupree, *Asa Gray 1810-1888* (Cambridge, 1959), 27; Lester S. King, *The Medical World of the Eighteenth Century* (Chicago, 1958), 193ff.

15. EJ, "Diary," I, 62b-62c, 118-19, CFPL; EJ, "Autobiography," 18-22, HLHU; Harvard College bills in EJ Papers, CFPL.

16. EJ, "Diary," I, 67-90, CFPL; EJ, "Autobiography," 11-14, HLHU.

17. EJ, "Diary," I, 92-96, 106, CFPL.

18. This dream is recounted in EJ, "Autobiography," 12-13, HLHU.

19. Understandably, Jarvis was especially attracted to those who behaved in orderly, predictable, and moral ways. See Jarvis's letter recommending Rev. Andrew P. Peabody for the presidency of Harvard College; his description was perhaps as applicable to himself as it was to Peabody (EJ to E.R. Hoar, December 6, 1859, EJLB, CLMHMS).

My understanding of Jarvis's compulsive personality has been enriched by reading Harry Stack Sullivan's *Clinical Studies in Psychiatry* (New York, 1956), chapter 12; David Shapiro's *Neurotic Styles*

(New York, 1965), chapter 2; and Leon Salzman's *The Obsessive Personality: Origins, Dynamics and Therapy* (New York, 1968).

20. EJ, "Diary," I, 129, 165, 183-84, CFPL; EJ, "Autobiography," 34-35, HLHU.

21. EJ, "Diary," I, 120-28, 141, 151, CFPL.

22. EJ, "Diary," I, 179-81, CFPL; EJ, "Autobiography," 30, HLHU; EJ, "Traditions and Reminiscences," 207ff., CFPL. Unfortunately the surviving sources do not reveal the nature of his speech impediment.

23. EJ, "Diary," I, 180-81, CFPL.

24. For an analysis of the medical profession and medical education see the following: Charles E. Rosenberg, "The American Medical Profession: Mid-Nineteenth Century," *Mid-America*, XLIV (July 1962), 163-71, and *The Cholera Years: The United States in 1832, 1849, and 1866* (Chicago, 1962); Joseph F. Kett, *The Formation of the American Medical Profession: The Role of Institutions, 1780-1860* (New Haven, 1968); Richard H. Shryock, *Medicine and Society in America 1660-1860* (New York, 1960); William G. Rothstein, *American Physicians in the Nineteenth Century: From Sects to Science* (Baltimore, 1972).

25. Grindall Reynolds, "Memoir of Dr. Josiah Bartlett," in *Memoirs of the Social Circle in Concord: Second Series*, 172-87; EJ, "Diary," I, 120, CFPL.

26. EJ, "Diary," I, 145, 159, 166, 174-76, CFPL; EJ, "Autobiography," 31, HLHU.

27. Thomas F. Harrington, *The Harvard Medical School: A History, Narrative and Documentary* (3 vols.: New York, 1905), passim; William F. Norwood, *Medical Education in the United States before the Civil War* (Philadelphia, 1944), 167-85; Morison, *Three Centuries of Harvard*, 167-73, 222-24. For a contemporary analysis see N. S. Davis, *History of Medical Education and Institutions in the United States from the First Settlement of the British Colonies to the Year 1850* (Chicago, 1851).

28. EJ, "Autobiography," 38, HLHU; EJ, "Diary," I, 195-96, 400-6, CFPL.

29. A self-limited disease, Bigelow wrote in his classic essay, was one "which receives limits from its own nature and not from foreign influences; one which, after it has obtained foothold in the system, cannot, in the present state of our knowledge, be eradicated or abridged by art, but to which there is due a certain succession of processes to be completed in a certain time; which time and processes may vary with the constitution and condition of the patient, and may tend

to death or to recovery, but are not known to be shortened or greatly changed by medical treatment.'' This essay first appeared in the *Medical Communications of the Massachusetts Medical Society*, V (1830–1836), 319–58.

30. Leonard K. Eaton, *New England Hospitals 1790–1833* (Ann Arbor, 1957), 169–71; Eleanor M. Tilton, *Amiable Autocrat: A Biography of Dr. Oliver Wendell Holmes* (New York, 1947), 76–79. The transitional nature of the curriculum was evident in Channing's course on midwifery, which Jarvis took during his first winter in Boston. See EJ, mss. notebook on Dr. Walter Channing, Jr., lectures on midwifery and medical jurisprudence in 1827–1828, CLMHMS.

31. EJ, "Diary," I, 177, 196, 200, 207–9, CFPL.

32. Ibid., 236–37; EJ, "Autobiography," 40–41, HLHU.

33. Willard Parker to EJ, July 10, 1828, EJ Papers, CLMHMS; EJ, "Diary," I, 261–62, CFPL.

34. Benjamin Lincoln to EJ, August 12, 16, 1828, EJ Papers, CLMHMS; EJ, "Diary," I, 262–303, CFPL.

35. *A Catalogue of the Officers and Students of Harvard University, for the Academical Year 1829-30* (Cambridge, 1829), 28–29; EJ, *Memoir of the Life and Character of George Cheyne Shattuck, M.D.* (n.p., c. 1854), 2; EJ, "Diary," I, 345, CFPL.

36. Shattuck's reputation, Jarvis recalled in 1854, was not due to any scientific qualities, for he did not aim ''at the highest scholarship in the science of his calling, nor at the most thoroughly disciplined exactness in his investigations of morbid symptoms.'' Shattuck's conclusions ''were rather the results of a sort of intuition than the cautiously drawn deductions of reason.'' See EJ, *Memoir of . . . George Cheyne Shattuck*, 2.

37. EJ, "Diary," I, 315–16, 341–47, CFPL; EJ, "Autobiography," 42, HLHU; EJ, *Memoir of . . . George Cheyne Shattuck*, 2–3.

38. EJ, "Diary," I, 348, 353–56, CFPL; EJ, "Autobiography," 43–44, HLHU.

39. EJ, "Diary," I, 212–16, 318, 323–29, 334–35, CFPL; EJ annotated notes to Lemuel Shattuck's *History of the Town of Concord* to be found between 190–91, copy in CFPL.

40. EJ, "Diary," I, 390–97, CFPL.

41. Ibid., 398–99. A copy of Jarvis's "Dissertation on Puerperal Fever" can be found in his mss. notebook on Dr. Walter Channing, Jr., lectures on midwifery and medical jurisprudence in 1827–1828, CLMHMS.

42. EJ, mss. notebook on Dr. Walter Channing, Jr., lectures on midwifery and medical jurisprudence in 1827–1828, 138–40, 157,

CLMHMS; EJ, "Diary," I, 348, 409–11, CFPL; EJ, "Autobiography," 49, HLHU; *Quinquennial Catalogue of the Officers and Graduates of Harvard University 1636-1905* (Cambridge, 1905), 354.

CHAPTER 2

1. EJ, "Diary" (2 mss. vols., 1827–1842), I, 416–23, CFPL; EJ, "Autobiography," 50–53, mss., HLHU.

2. EJ, "Diary," I, 424, II, 1–9, CFPL; EJ, "Autobiography," 54–57, HLHU.

3. EJ, "Diary," II, 28–30, 72, CFPL.

4. EJ, "Autobiography," 57–59, HLHU; EJ, "Diary," II, 26, CFPL.

5. EJ to Benjamin Lincoln, September 13, 1832, Lincoln Papers, CLMHMS; EJ, "Diary," II, 15, 19, 21, 24–26, 43, 51, 72, 86–88, CFPL.

6. EJ to Benjamin Lincoln, July 22, 1833, Lincoln Papers, CLMHMS. See also EJ, "Autobiography," 44–48, HLHU.

7. EJ to Benjamin Lincoln, May 22 and June 23, 1832, May 2 and July 22, 1833, Lincoln Papers, CLMHMS; EJ, "Diary," II, 55–56, 61–62, 86, CFPL.

Jarvis's experiences made him all the more sympathetic to the plight of his former teacher, Benjamin Lincoln, who became embroiled in a public controversy over medical education and religion in Vermont in the early 1830s. In Lincoln's situation Jarvis may have seen a reflection of his own. Both men were seeking to elevate humanity; their enemies were unprincipled and unscrupulous men seeking only partisan and narrow self-interest. "Is not the world's gullibility its greatest quality?" asked Jarvis in a letter to Lincoln. "I did not believe it at first, but many proofs have wrought a sad change in my faith. Tis not he who knows the most, but he that makes the widest pretensions & most accommodates himself & his science to the ignorance & preconceptions of the world, that prospers most among feeble mortality." See EJ to Benjamin Lincoln, May 22, June 23, and September 15, 1832, May 2, 1833, Lincoln Papers, CLMHMS. The controversy can be followed in Lincoln's *Hints on the Present State of Medical Education and the Influence of Medical Schools in New England* (Burlington, 1833), and Lester J. Wallman, "Benjamin Lincoln, M.D. Vermont Medical Educator," *Vermont History,* XXIX (October 1961), 196–209.

8. EJ, "Diary," II, 15, 20, 28, 31, 66, CFPL; EJ to Benjamin Lincoln, May 22 and June 23, 1832, Lincoln Papers, CLMHMS. The Jarvis papers do not contain Lincoln's reply (if any).

9. EJ, "Account of a Remarkable Epidemic in Warwick, Mass.,"*Medical Magazine,* I (February 1833), 449-54. For an analysis about dominant medical thinking about cholera in the early 1830s see Charles E. Rosenberg, *The Cholera Years: The United States in 1832, 1849, and 1866* (Chicago, 1962), 65-81.

10. EJ, "Diary," II, 68-71, 73-84, CFPL.

11. Ibid., 93-96.

12. Ibid., 96-108, 117-22; EJ to Benjamin Lincoln, May 2, 1833, Lincoln Papers, CLMHMS.

13. EJ, "Diary," II, 96-100, 112-14, 117, 119-21, 123, 130-31, 136-41, CFPL.

14. Ibid., 131-34; EJ, "Autobiography," 70-75, HLHU; *Concord Freeman,* January 9, 1836; *Yeoman's Gazette* (Concord), January 16, 1836; EJ to Henry J. Hosmer, March 16, 1882, in *The Centennial of the Social Circle in Concord March 21, 1882* (Cambridge, 1882), 44-45; EJ, "Traditions and Reminiscences of Concord Massachusetts, or a Contribution to the Social and Domestic History of the Town from 1779 to 1878," mss. vol., CFPL (see especially 331-33); Mss. Records of the Concord Lyceum, Recording Secretary, vol. I (1828-1859), 69, 72-78, 81-82, 86-87, 89-91, 98-101, 103, 107, 115, 121, 125, 131, CFPL. Jarvis also knew Ralph Waldo Emerson sufficiently well to ask the latter if he could read his journal which he kept during a trip to Europe. See EJ to Emerson, June 28, 1834, Ralph Waldo Emerson Papers, HLHU. Emerson's response apparently has not survived.

15. EJ, "Ladies' Fairs," *New England Magazine,* V (July 1833), 54-59; EJ, "Autobiography," 74, HLHU.

16. EJ, "Autobiography," 79-81, HLHU.

17. Based on the epistemological theory advanced by the Abbé Étienne de Condillac, the philosophy of Ideology was further developed by Destutt de Tracy, Helvétius, Condorcet, Cabanis, and others. According to Condillac, sensations were the primary data of cognition. All ideas and all the faculties of human understanding, furthermore, were simply compounds of sensations that could be resolved by an analytical method into their component parts. The basis of all ideas, in other words, was experience; nothing could be present in the mind except what entered it through the senses. To Condillac's disciples, this method of radical empiricism was crucial. Not only would it enable man to learn and understand his nature, but he would be able to undertake a political, social, economic, and moral reconstruction in order to better his condition. See George Rosen, "The Philosophy of Ideology and the Emergence of Modern Medicine

in France," *Bulletin of the History of Medicine,* XX (July 1946), 328-31.

18. See George Rosen, "Problems in the Application of Statistical Analysis to Questions of Health: 1700-1880," *Bulletin of the History of Medicine,* XXIX (January–February 1955), 27-45; Richard H. Shryock, *The Development of Modern Medicine: An Interpretation of the Social and Scientific Factors Involved* (rev. ed., New York, 1947), 157-69; Major Greenwood, *Medical Statistics from Graunt to Farr* (Cambridge, England, 1948).

19. EJ, "Autobiography," 47-48, HLHU.

20. EJ, "Concord to Louisville 1837" (a journal), 93, mss. in CLMHMS; EJ, "Diary," I, 250, CFPL.

21. EJ, "Intemperance and Disease," *Boston Medical and Surgical Journal,* XV (November 30, 1836), 261-67; EJ, "Traditions and Reminiscences," 445-50, CFPL; Mss. Records of the Concord Lyceum, Recording Secretary, vol. I, 75, CFPL; *Yeoman's Gazette,* June 25, 1836; EJ, *Financial Connection of the Use of Spirits and Wine with the People of Concord, Massachusetts* (Boston, 1883), 5-8.

22. EJ, "Diary," II, 138-39, CFPL; EJ, "Autobiography," 77-78, HLHU.

23. For discussions of nineteenth-century American psychiatric thought and practice see Norman Dain, *Concepts of Insanity in the United States, 1789-1865* (New Brunswick, 1964), and Gerald N. Grob, *Mental Institutions in America: Social Policy to 1875* (New York, 1973), and *The State and the Mentally Ill: A History of Worcester State Hospital in Massachusetts 1830-1920* (Chapel Hill, 1966).

24. Cf. EJ, "Insanity in Kentucky," *Boston Medical and Surgical Journal,* XXIV (April 21, 1841), 165-71, and his review article on insanity and insane asylums in the *Western Journal of Medicine and Surgery,* IV (December 1841), 443-82.

25. EJ to Dr. Benjamin Barrett, January 30, 1857, EJLB, CLMHMS.

26. Ralph Waldo Emerson to Josiah Quincy, Jr., December 10, 1836, in *The Letters of Ralph Waldo Emerson,* ed. Ralph L. Rusk (6 vols.: New York, 1939), II, 49-50; EJ, "Diary," II, 144-47, CFPL; EJ, "Autobiography," 78-79, HLHU.

27. EJ, "Diary," II, 153, CFPL; EJ, "Autobiography," 82, HLHU.

28. EJ, "Concord to Louisville 1837" (a journal), 1-45, mss. in CLMHMS. It should be noted that the Rev. Louis Dwight (whom Jarvis believed had blocked his appointment as superintendent of McLean some months before) was the leading opponent of the Pennsylvania

prison reformers. Jarvis's affinity for the latter may have partially reflected some of his hostility toward Dwight.

29. Ibid., 47–134.

30. Ibid., 135–70.

31. Information on Louisville culled from Ben Casseday, *The History of Louisville, from its Earliest Settlement Till the Year 1852* (Louisville, 1852); Richard C. Wade, *The Urban Frontier: The Rise of Western Cities, 1790-1830* (Cambridge, 1959); and Josiah Stoddard Johnston, *Memorial History of Louisville from its First Settlement to the Year 1896* (2 vols.: Chicago, 1896).

32. EJ, "Diary" (2 mss. vols., 1827–1842), II, 177–78, CFPL; EJ, "Autobiography," 84–89, mss., HLHU.

33. EJ to James Jackson (2 letters), September 25, 1837, Jackson Papers, CLMHMS.

34. Louisville *Daily Journal,* January 20, March 10, 18, 29, April 1, 5, 10, 22, May 3, 6, 9, 26, 1837; Charles Caldwell, *Autobiography of Charles Caldwell, M.D.,* ed. Harriot W. Warner (Philadelphia, 1855), 399ff.; Hampden C. Lawson, "The Early Medical Schools of Kentucky," *Bulletin of the History of Medicine,* XXIV (March–April 1950), 168–71; William F. Norwood, *Medical Education in the United States before the Civil War* (Philadelphia, 1944), 289–301; Madge E. Pickard and R. Carlyle Buley, *The Midwest Pioneer: His Ills, Cures, & Doctors* (New York, 1946), 120ff.; Medical Historical Research Project of the Works Projects Administration, *Medicine and its Development in Kentucky* (Louisville, 1940), chap. 6.

35. Louisville *Daily Journal,* May 18, 19, 20, 21, 22, 23, 25, 26, 30, June 13, 1840; Lawson, "The Early Medical Schools of Kentucky," 170–71; EJ, "Autobiography," 92–94, HLHU; Willard Parker to EJ, August 20, 1838, EJ Papers, CLMHMS.

36. EJ, "True Delicacy Toward Animals," *Western Messenger,* VI (November 1838), 19–24; idem., "Mr. Young's Discourse on the Life and Character of Dr. Bowditch," ibid., VI (November 1838), 63–66; and idem., "New-England Non-Resistance Society," ibid., VIII (September 1840), 193–201.

37. EJ, letter (written September 17, 1838) to the *Yeoman's Gazette* (Concord), November 24, 1838.

38. EJ, "Autobiography," 98–99, HLHU; EJ to Horace Mann, February 25, 1840, Mann Papers, MHS; Johnston, *Memorial History of Louisville,* I, 234–35.

39. EJ, "Sixth Annual Report of the Board of Education. With the Sixth Annual Report of the Secretary of the Board" (review of Horace

Mann's reports), *Christian Examiner*, XXXIV (July 1843), 367. See also EJ to Mann, February 25, 1840, and February 9 and March 15, 1842, Mann Papers, MHS.

Shortly after leaving Louisville Jarvis condemned the prominence of males in the teaching profession. Too many men refused to make teaching a permanent career, thereby vitiating their effectiveness. Since the role of the teacher was vital, Jarvis urged more widespread employment of females at wages equal to those paid their male counterparts. See EJ, "Sixth Annual Report of the Board of Education," 370–77.

40. EJ to Horace Mann, February 9 and March 15, 1842, Mann Papers, MHS; Louisville *Daily Journal,* May 13, 16, 18 and June 7, 8, 1842; Theodore S. Bell to EJ, May 7, 1843, EJ Papers, CLMHMS.

Jarvis was also the driving force in establishing the Kentucky Historical Society in 1838 and helped to amass a large collection of printed materials; knowledge of the past, after all, was vital for future enlightenment. The society became defunct after he left Louisville. See EJ, "Some Account of the Kentucky Historical Society," *American Quarterly Register*, XV (August 1842), 72–77; EJ, "Kentucky Historical Society," *Western Messenger*, VI (November 1838), 61–62; Louisville *Daily Journal*, February 26, 1839, January 22, 1840; Theodore S. Bell to EJ, May 7, 1843, EJ Papers, CLMHMS.

As in Concord, Jarvis often gave lectures in Louisville. See the Louisville *Daily Journal*, October 31, 1839, February 15, 1840, February 5, 1841.

41. Kentucky Eastern Lunatic Asylum, *Annual Report*, 1844, 19–21; Gerald N. Grob, *Mental Institutions in America: Social Policy to 1875* (New York, 1973), 343–44; Samuel Theobold, "Some Account of the Lunatic Asylum of Kentucky, with Remarks, &c.," *Transylvania Journal of Medicine and the Associate Sciences* II (November 1829), 500–11, III (February 1830), 79–94.

42. Some of the psychiatric literature published before 1840 reflected a casualness about detail that may have been partly a function of the unavailability of material. Amariah Brigham's article in the *North American Review* in 1837 included numerous errors, a fact noted by Jarvis in his article. Brigham, for example, gave Kentucky credit for founding the first public hospital in 1824 and ignored Virginia; he also gave 1812 rather than 1830 as the date of the founding of the Worcester hospital in Massachusetts. See Brigham, "Insanity and Insane Hospitals," *North American Review*, XLIV (January 1837), 91–121.

43. EJ, "Insanity in Kentucky," *Boston Medical and Surgical Journal*, XXIV (April 21, 1841), 165–71.

44. EJ, review article in the *Western Journal of Medicine and Surgery*, IV (December 1841), 443–82, also circulated in pamphlet form under the title *Insanity and Insane Asylums* (Louisville, 1841).

45. EJ, "What Shall We Do with Our Insane?," *Western Journal of Medicine and Surgery*, V (February 1842), 81–125, also circulated in pamphlet form under the title *What Shall We Do with the Insane of the Western Country?* (Louisville, 1842).

46. Louisville *Daily Journal*, November 30 and December 9, 1841; EJ, "Insane Asylums in the West," *Boston Medical and Surgical Journal*, XXVI (March 23, 1842), 101–6; EJ letter on "Prospects of the Blind and Insane in Kentucky," *Boston Medical and Surgical Journal*, XXVI (March 2, 1842), 60–61, 63.

47. EJ to Horace Mann, March 15, 1842, Mann Papers, MHS; EJ, "Autobiography," 118–19, HLHU; EJ, "Diary," II, 179–81, CFPL; Kentucky Eastern Lunatic Asylum, *Annual Report*, 1844, 19–31; ibid., 1869, 11–14; *Boston Medical and Surgical Journal*, XXXI (December 11, 1844), 386.

48. Louisville *Daily Journal*, February 5, 8, 9, 19 and March 8, 14, 1842; EJ, letter on "Prospects of the Blind and Insane in Kentucky," *Boston Medical and Surgical Journal*, XXVI (March 2, 1842), 60–61; *Western Journal of Medicine and Surgery*, V (April, 1842), 317–19; EJ, "Autobiography," 119–20, HLHU. For other examples of Jarvis's benevolent activities see EJ, "Autobiography," 94–97, 108–11, HLHU; EJ, "Diary," II, 169–71, CFPL.

49. EJ, letter to *Yeoman's Gazette* (Concord), February 24, 1838 (letter dated January 1838); EJ, "Autobiography," 109–11, 122–23, HLHU; EJ, "Diary," II, 175–76, CFPL; EJ, "Journal of a Journey from Louisville to New Orleans of a Visit of Eight Days in New Orleans. And Return to Louisville Ky April 16th to May 6th, 1841," mss., CFPL.

50. EJ, "Diary," II, 177–78, CFPL; EJ to Francis E. Goddard, July 28, 1843, EJLB, CLMHMS.

51. EJ, "Diary," II, 189, CFPL.

52. EJ to Horace Mann, February 9, March 15, 1842, Mann Papers, MHS.

53. EJ to Samuel B. Woodward, April 11, 1842; Woodward to EJ, April 18, 1842; James Jackson to EJ, May 30 and July 9, 1842; Charles B. Coventry to EJ, June 14, 1842, EJ Papers, CLMHMS.

54. EJ, "Diary," II, 184, 188–91, CFPL.

CHAPTER 3

1. Cf. EJ's "Traditions and Reminiscences of Concord Massachusetts, or a Contribution to the Social and Domestic History of the Town 1779 to 1878," mss. vol., CFPL.
2. Frank H. Hankins, *Adolphe Quetelet as Statistician* (New York, 1908), 60.
3. EJ, "Autobiography," 124–26, mss., HLHU.
4. EJ to Samuel Gridley Howe, November 5, 1842, Howe Papers, HLHU (HLHU incorrectly lists the date of this letter as 1845); George Sumner to EJ, March 20, 1843, EJ Papers, CLMHMS; EJ, "Autobiography," 126–29, HLHU. For evidence of Woodward's connection with the Hartford Retreat see Woodward to George Sumner, March 18, 1834, and Thomas H. Gallandet to Woodward, February 21, 1840, Woodward Papers, AAS.
5. George Sumner to Luther V. Bell, March 13, 1843, and Luther V. Bell to Isaac Ray, n.d. (March 1843) (appended to Sumner letter), Isaac Ray Medical Library, Butler Hospital, Providence, R.I. Sumner's letter indicated strong support for Ray's candidacy. Bell then forwarded this letter to Ray with the comment about Jarvis and also expressing surprise that Butler was being considered for the position "in face of his long continued ill success" in Boston.
6. EJ, "Autobiography," 129–32, HLHU; EJ, "The Late Dr. Robert Thaxter, of Dorchester," *Boston Medical and Surgical Journal*, XLVI (May 19, 1852), 309–14.
7. EJ to Eveline Blodgett, April 4, 1849, EJ to James Dixon, April 18, 1853, EJ to Mary G. Hopkins, August 8, 1854, EJ to Thomas S. Kirkbride, July 21, 1855, EJ to William Ingalls, April 2, 1856, EJ to Edward Hallester, September 23, 1856, EJ to John W. Green, November 18, 1856, EJ to B. Scheifferlin, April 14, 1857, EJ to William A. Gorden, October 19, 1861, EJ to J. B. Chetwood, March 18, 1864, EJ to Thomas M. Cutter, August 7, 1866, EJLB, CLMHMS; Samuel Jackson to EJ, July 21, 1844, Luther V. Bell to EJ, April 7, 1849, Willard Parker to EJ, April 30, May 3, 24, June 19, 1855, EJ Papers, CLMHMS; EJ, "Autobiography," 137–38, HLHU.
8. EJ to John Abbott, February 11, 1850, EJ to H. Cowperthwait & Co., August 9, 1858, EJ to Josephine C.B. Nourse, August 26, September 14, 22, 25, October 6, 9, 12, 13, 16, 1857, April 17, June 7, 1858, EJ to James B. Murch, March 10, July 22, October 25, November 3, 1859, EJ to William B. Heiskell, March 5, June 5, 1859, EJ to William G. Ladd, December 24, 1862, May 22, 1865, EJ to Alexander Holmes, April 7, 1864, EJ to A. W. Draper, January 22, 1866, EJ to

William M. Pritchard, October 19, 1866, August 16, 1869, EJ to Francis C. Barlow, December 23, 1867, EJ to James M. Keith, May 21, 1872, EJ to William Withington, May 7, 1874, May 3, 1878, EJLB, CLMHMS; Luther V. Bell to EJ, July 8, 1853, EJ Papers, CLMHMS; EJ, "Autobiography," 139, HLHU; EJ Will and Almira Jarvis Will (Nos. 72,319 and 72,320), Suffolk County Probate Court, Boston, Mass.

9. EJ to Charlotte M. Haven, December 5, 1860, EJ to Eveline Blodgett, April 4, 1849, EJLB, CLMHMS; EJ, "Autobiography," 138, HLHU; "Edward Jarvis," *American Academy of Arts and Sciences, Proceedings,* n.s. XII (1884–1885), 521.

10. Isaac Ray to EJ, July 2, 1859, John S. Butler to EJ, July 4, 1859, EJ Papers, CLMHMS; EJ to George Chandler, April 12, 1856, EJ to George C.S. Choate, April 12, 1856, EJ to J.B. Chetwood, March 18, 1864, EJLB, CLMHMS; EJ, "Autobiography," 138, 141, HLHU.

11. EJ, "Law of Physical Life," *Christian Examiner,* XXXV (September 1843), 1–31. The first article was entitled "Sixth Annual Report of the Board of Education With the Sixth Annual Report of the Secretary of the Board," ibid., XXXIV (July 1843), 366–81.

12. Charles G. Putnam to EJ, December 16, 1848, EJ Papers, CLMHMS.

13. EJ, "The Production of Vital Force," in *Medical Communications of the Massachusetts Medical Society,* 2d ser. IV (Boston, 1854), 1–40.

14. There was a favorable review of Jarvis's address in the *American Journal of the Medical Sciences,* n.s. XX (July 1850), 156–59, and Jacob Bigelow spoke well of it, although he urged Jarvis to keep details to a minimum. See Bigelow to EJ, July 11, 1849, EJ Papers, CLMHMS.

15. EJ, notations on letter from Josiah Bartlett to EJ, October 29, 1848, EJ Papers, CLMHMS.

16. Cf. Thomas S. Kuhn's *The Structure of Scientific Revolutions* (Chicago, 1962).

17. Cf. John C. Warren, "New Theory of Human Deformity," *Boston Medical and Surgical Journal,* III (November 9, 1830), 642, cited in George H. Daniels, *American Science in the Age of Jackson* (New York, 1968), 66; William M. Awl to Samuel B. Woodward, April 18, 1842, Woodward Papers, AAS.

18. Lester S. King, *The Medical World of the Eighteenth Century* (Chicago, 1958), chap. 7.

19. This analysis of mid-nineteenth-century American science is based upon Daniels, *American Science in the Age of Jackson,* 66–67, 102, 144–45, et passim.

20. Cf. "The Approaching Census," *United States Magazine and*

Democratic Review, V (January 1839), 77–85. For background material on the history of the censuses see the following: Walter F. Willcox, *Studies in American Demography* (Ithaca, 1940), chap. 4; W. Stull Holt, *The Bureau of the Census: Its History, Activities and Organization* (Washington, D.C., 1929), chap. 1; Carroll D. Wright and William C. Hunt, *The History and Growth of the United States Census* (Washington, D.C., 1900), passim.

21. The raw data on this subject can be found in the *Compendium of the Enumeration of the Inhabitants and Statistics of the United States, as Obtained at the Department of State, from the Returns of the Sixth Census* (Washington, D.C., 1841), 4–103. I have used the ratios, which are generally accurate, computed by Jarvis in his article "Insanity Among the Coloured Population of the Free States," *American Journal of the Medical Sciences,* n.s. VII (January 1844), 72–73.

22. Virginia Western Lunatic Asylum, *Annual Report,* XIV (1841), 38–43; C.B. Hayden, "On the Distribution of Insanity in the U. States," *Southern Literary Messenger,* X (March 1844), 180; *The Works of John C. Calhoun,* ed. Richard K. Crallé (6 vols.: New York, 1870–1876), V, 333–39. For other reactions see the following: "Statistics of Population. Table of Lunacy in the United States," *Hunt's Merchants' Magazine,* VIII (March 1843), 290, and "Table of Lunacy in the United States," ibid., VIII (May 1843), 460–61; "Reflections on the Census of 1840," *Southern Literary Messenger,* IX (June 1843), 340–52; Samuel Forrey, "Vital Statistics Furnished by the Sixth Census of the United States, Bearing upon the Question of the Unity of the Human Race," and "On the Relative Proportion of Centenarians, of Deaf and Dumb, of Blind, and of Insane, in the Races of European and African Origin, as Shown by the Censuses of the United States," *New York Journal of Medicine and the Collateral Sciences,* I (September 1843), 151–67; ibid., II (May 1844), 310–20.

23. EJ, "Statistics of Insanity in the United States," *Boston Medical and Surgical Journal,* XXVII (September 21, 1842), 116–21.

24. EJ, "Statistics of Insanity in the United States," ibid., XXVII (November 30, 1842), 281–82.

25. EJ, "Insanity Among the Coloured Population of the Free States," *American Journal of the Medical Sciences,* n.s. VII (January 1844), 71–83; *Western Journal of Medicine and Surgery,* n.s. I (February 1844), 181–82.

26. Henry I. Bowditch to EJ, undated letter (c. 1843) and January 19, 1844, EJ Papers, CLMHMS; "Records of the American Statistical Asso-

ciation 1839-1872," mss. vol., 23-24, ASA; *Medical Communications of the Massachusetts Medical Society,* VII (1842-1848), Appendix, 59, 67, 72, 83-84, 90-95; EJ to Dorothea L. Dix, May 25, 1844, Dix Papers, HLHU.

27. 28th Cong., 1st Sess., *Journal of the House of Representatives,* 471, 877, 932-33, 1170; 28th Cong., 1st Sess., *House Document No. 245* (May 4, 1844); 28th Cong., 1st Sess., *House Report No. 580* (June 17, 1844).

28. 28th Cong., 1st Sess., *House Report No. 579* (June 17, 1844), *House Report No. 580* (June 17, 1844); 28th Cong., 2d Sess., *Journal of the House of Representatives,* 291, 369, *Journal of the Senate,* 27, 30, 214, *Senate Document No. 5* (December 10, 1844), *Senate Document No. 146* (February 27, 1845), *House Document No. 116* (February 12, 1845), *Congressional Globe,* December 16, 1844, 17-18.

29. EJ, J. Wingate Thornton, and William Brigham, "The Sixth Census of the United States," *Hunt's Merchants' Magazine,* XII (February 1845), 125-39; *Boston Medical and Surgical Journal,* XXX (June 5, 1844), 362-63; *American Journal of Insanity,* I (July 1844), 78-81; *Western Journal of Medicine and Surgery,* n.s. I (February 1844), 181-82; Pliny Earle to EJ, May 11, 1844, and Samuel B. Woodward to EJ, September 14, 1844, EJ Papers, CLMHMS; EJ to John Gorham Palfrey, January 30, 1849 (HLHU erroneously lists date as 1844), Palfrey Papers, HLHU; EJ to Charles Sumner, February 13, 1852, Sumner Papers, HLHU; EJ to J.D.B. De Bow, January 18, 30, 1854, EJ to Joseph C.G. Kennedy, August 26, 1859, EJ to Charles Sumner, December 31, 1867, EJLB, CLMHMS; "Startling Facts from the Census," *American Journal of Insanity,* VIII (October 1851), 153-55; EJ, "Insanity Among the Coloured Population of the Free States," *American Journal of Insanity,* VIII (January 1852), 268-82; EJ, "Autobiography," 134-37, HLHU.

30. "Records of the American Statistical Association 1839-1872," 35-36, 38, 42-43, ASA; EJ and Committee of the American Statistical Association to Senator William L. Dayton, August 30, 1848, EJLB, CLMHMS; EJ to John Gorham Palfrey, January 30, 1849, Palfrey Papers, HLHU.

31. EJ to Horace Mann, November 23, 1842, Mann Papers, MHS; EJ to Nahum Capen and William B. Fowler, May 13, June 27, 1843, EJLB, CLMHMS. Capen was a popularizer of phrenology in the United States.

32. EJ, *Lecture on the Necessity of the Study of Physiology, Delivered Before the American Institute of Instruction, at Hartford,*

August 22, 1845 (Boston, 1845), passim. See the favorable review in the *American Journal of the Medical Sciences,* n.s. XI (April 1846), 435–36.

33. EJ to Thomas, Cowperthwait, & Co., May 19, August 28, 1847, EJ to David M. Warren, July 20, 1847, EJ to John C. Warren, December, 1847, April 28, 1848, EJ to Horace Mann, August 24, 1853, EJ to Joseph B. Cowperthwait, August 27, 1862, EJLB, CLMHMS; EJ to John C. Warren, April 28, May 30, 1848, Warren Papers, MHS.

34. EJ, *Practical Physiology; For the Use of Schools and Families* (Philadelphia, 1847), 351–52, 367.

35. Ibid., 23ff., 86–87. This work went through several different editions, most of which were simply reprintings. In 1852 the book— slightly revised and with seventy new engravings—was issued under the title *Practical Physiology; Or, Anatomy and Physiology Applied to Health, for the Use of Schools and Families* (Philadelphia, 1852).

36. See EJ to T. Southwood Smith, June 10, 1850, EJLB, CLMHMS. Jarvis was referring to Smith's *The Philosophy of Health* (2 vols.: London, 1835–1837).

37. *American Journal of the Medical Sciences,* n.s. XV (January 1848), 212–13.

38. EJ, *Primary Physiology, for Schools* (Philadelphia, 1848); EJ to Thomas, Cowperthwait, & Co., February 3, May 31, 1848, EJ to Charles Brooks, August 14, 1848, EJLB, CLMHMS. See the favorable notice in the *Boston Medical and Surgical Journal,* XXXIX (September 6, 1848), 125.

39. "Report of the Annual Visiting Committees of the Public Schools of the City of Boston, 1847," Boston *City Document No. 40* (1847), 39–45, 63; George B. Emerson, "Report on Books," Boston *City Document No. 21* (1847), 2–7; Calvin Cutter, *First Book on Anatomy and Physiology* (Boston, 1848), 128–32, et passim; EJ to Thomas, Cowperthwait & Co., July 26, 1848, EJLB, CLMHMS. Subsequently Cutter published a longer work under the title *A Treatise on Anatomy, Physiology, and Hygiene: Designed for Colleges, Academies, and Families* (Boston, 1850).

40. EJ to Charles Brooks, August 14, 1848, EJ to Thomas, Cowperthwait, & Co., August 9, September 25, October 5, 1848, EJ to Charles Northend, July 28, 1848, EJLB, CLMHMS.

41. "The Report of the Annual Examination of the Public Schools of the City of Boston. 1848," Boston *City Document No. 31* (1848), 25; "The Report of the Annual Examination of the Public Schools of the City of Boston. 1849," Boston *City Document No. 39* (1849), 16, 20–22; "The Report of the Annual Examination of the Public Schools

of the City of Boston. 1850," Boston *City Document No. 38* (1850), 5, 7, 9–10, 18–19; EJ to John Codman, November 19, 1849, EJ to Thomas, Cowperthwait, & Co., January 31, August 8, 1850, EJLB, CLMHMS.

42. EJ to Horace Mann, August 24, 1853, EJ to Thomas, Cowperthwait, & Co., April 18, August 23, 1853, February 15, 1854, EJ to Cowperthwait, Desilver & Co., August 8, 1854, EJ to H. Cowperthwait & Co., February 1, 1856, January 3, 1857, EJLB, CLMHMS.

43. EJ to Samuel Gridley Howe, August 27, 1862, EJ to Joseph Cowperthwait, August 27, 1862, February 4, 1864, EJ to William B. Haskell, May 26, June 8, July 20, August 11, 16, 1864, EJ to Robert S. Davis, February 8, 1865, EJ to Barnes & Burr, July 13, 1865, EJ to A.S. Barnes & Co., July 26, August 3, September 4, 18, 26, 1865, April 13, May ?, August 17, September 1, October 12, 1866, January 19, July 20, 1867, January 23, July 18, 1868, January 21, 1869, January 21, 29, 1870, January 23, July 24, 1871, January 22, 1872, July 20, 1874, August 8, November 23, December 23, 27, 1876, January 24, 1877, EJLB, CLMHMS; EJ, *Physiology and Laws of Health. For the Use of Schools, Academies, and Colleges* (New York, 1866), and *Primary Physiology* (New York, 1866).

In 1881 Jarvis's book was translated into Chinese by a Methodist firm, presumably for the use of missionaries. See EJ to James Magee, March 18, 1881, EJLB, CLMHMS. There is a copy of the Chinese edition in the CLMHMS.

44. EJ, "Plan of a course of lectures," included with a letter from EJ to B.E. Cotting, July 29, 1854, EJLB, CLMHMS.

CHAPTER 4

1. *Medical Communications of the Massachusetts Medical Society,* 2d ser. I (Boston, 1836), Appendix, 69; ibid., 2d ser. III (Boston, 1848), Appendix, 47–48, 72, 153, 162–63; ibid., 2d ser. IV (Boston, 1854), Proceedings, 3, 5, 15, 22, 30, 65, 78, 142; Walter L. Burrage, *A History of the Massachusetts Medical Society . . . 1781–1922* (Norwood, 1923), 149–50, 296, 428–31.

2. These generalizations are based on the following sources: "Records of the American Statistical Association 1839–1872," "Record Book. American Statistical Association, 1872–1916," "Records of the Board of Directors of the American Statistical Association in Boston," mss. vols., ASA; EJ, "Autobiography," mss. vol., 325–26, HLHU.

3. This paragraph is based on R.A. Lewis, *Edwin Chadwick and the*

Public Health Movement 1832–1854 (London, 1952), chaps. 1–2. See also S.E. Finer, *The Life and Times of Sir Edwin Chadwick* (London, 1952).

4. EJ, "Chadwick on the Practice of Interment in Towns," *American Journal of the Medical Sciences,* IX (January 1845), 131–54.

5. Ibid., 142–43, 152–53.

6. Robley Dunglison, *Human Health; or the Influence of Atmosphere and Locality; Change of Air and Climate; Seasons; Food; Clothing; Bathing and Mineral Springs; Exercise; Sleep; Corporeal and Intellectual Pursuits, &c., &c., on Healthy Man; Constituting Elements of Hygiene* (new ed.: Philadelphia, 1844).

7. EJ, "Dunglison on Human Health," *American Journal of the Medical Sciences,* n.s. IX (April 1845), 379–90.

8. See George Rosen, *A History of Public Health* (New York, 1958), 259–64.

9. Oliver Wendell Holmes to EJ, August 6, 1845, EJ Papers, CLMHMS; EJ to Isaac Hays, September 8, 1845, EJLB, CLMHMS; Thomas Laycock, "Notice of Some Vital Statistics of the United States, in a Letter to the Hon. Horace Mann, by Mr. Edward Jarvis, of Dorchester, Massachusetts, United States, dated 22nd April, 1845. Abstracted and Compared with the Statistics of England and Wales," *Journal of the Statistical Society of London,* IX (October 1846), 277–79 (this paper was read before the Statistical Section of the British Association on June 23, 1845). A copy of Jarvis's prize-winning dissertation does not seem to have survived.

10. See Robert Gutman, "Birth and Death Registration in Massachusetts. I. The Colonial Background, 1639–1800," *Milbank Memorial Fund Quarterly,* XXXVI (January 1958), 58–74, and "Birth and Death Registration in Massachusetts. II. The Inauguration of a Modern System, 1800–1849," ibid., XXXVI (October 1958), 373–402; James H. Cassedy, *Demography in Early America: Beginnings of the Statistical Mind, 1600–1800* (Cambridge, 1969); John B. Blake, "The Early History of Vital Statistics in Massachusetts," *Bulletin of the History of Medicine,* XXIX (January–February 1955), 46–68.

11. In justifying his presentation of aggregate data, Shattuck remarked that "few subjects are more interesting than accurate bills of mortality. They are the most authentic evidence of the influence of climate and local circumstances on health and human life; and teach a lesson, admonishing us of the destiny that awaits all mankind, and warning us 'to live prepared to die'" (Shattuck, *A History of the Town of Concord* [Boston, 1835], 223).

12. This discussion of Shattuck is based upon Barbara G. Rosenkrantz's *Public Health and the State: Changing Views in Massachusetts, 1842-1936* (Cambridge, 1972), 14-22. See also the following: Shattuck Papers, MHS; Shattuck, "The Vital Statistics of Boston from 1810-1841," *American Journal of the Medical Sciences,* n.s. I (April 1841), 369-400; idem., *Report to the Committee of the City Council Appointed to Obtain the Census of Boston for the Year 1845, Embracing Collateral Facts and Statistical Researches Illustrating the History and Conditions of the Population, and Their Means of Progress and Prosperity* (Boston, 1846).

13. EJ to Horace Mann, February 6, 1844, Mann Papers, MHS; Isaac Ray to EJ, July 3, 1844, EJ Papers, CLMHMS.

14. *Medical Communications of the Massachusetts Medical Society,* 2d ser. III (Boston, 1848), Appendix, 36, 47-61.

15. Ibid., 61-66.

16. *Proceedings of the National Medical Convention Held in New York, May, 1846, and in Philadelphia, May, 1847* (Philadelphia, 1847), 20-21.

17. Ibid., 37, 133-75. Griscom's report for the committee on registration can be found in ibid., 125-31.

18. This discussion of Farr is based upon John M. Eyler, "William Farr on the Cholera: The Sanitarian's Disease Theory and the Statistician's Method," *Journal of the History of Medicine and Allied Sciences,* XXVIII (April 1973), 79-100.

19. See particularly the "Memorial of Lemuel Shattuck, Praying for a Revision of the Laws in Relation to the Registration and Return of Births, Marriages, and Deaths," Mass. *Senate Document No. 24* (January 21, 1848), 32-33.

20. "Records of the American Statistical Association 1839-1872," 34-36, ASA; Lemuel Shattuck to EJ, February 11, 1848, EJ Papers, CLMHMS; EJ, "Autobiography," 186-87, HLHU.

21. Mass. *House Document No. 16* (February 9, 1848), 2-20.

22. EJ to John C. Warren, May 30, 1848, Warren Papers, MHS; *Medical Communications of the Massachusetts Medical Society,* 2d ser. III (Boston, 1848), 162-63; "Sanitary Survey of the State," Mass. *House Document No. 66* (March 3, 1849), 3-19; EJ, "Autobiography," 187-88, HLHU.

23. EJ, "Sanitary Reform," *American Journal of the Medical Sciences,* XV (April 1848), 419-50. In 1849 Jarvis published an article reviewing a number of treatises dealing with ventilation in which he related his general views to a specific problem. See EJ, "Treatises on Ventilation," ibid., n.s. XVIII (July 1849), 129-47.

24. Charles E. Rosenberg, "The Bitter Fruit: Heredity, Disease, and Social Thought in Nineteenth-Century America," *Perspectives in American History*, VIII (1974), 191–92.

25. Charles W. Wilder to EJ, January 23, 1849, EJ Papers, CLMHMS; EJ, "Report of the Sanitary Commission of Massachusetts," *Boston Medical and Surgical Journal*, XLIV (March 5, 1851), 89–90; Rosenkrantz, *Public Health and the State*, 28–29; Ray A. Billington, *The Protestant Crusade 1800–1860: A Study of the Origins of American Nativism* (New York, 1938), passim; Oscar Handlin, *Boston's Immigrants: A Study in Acculturation* (rev. ed.: Cambridge, 1959), passim.

26. *Report of the Special Joint Committee of the Legislature of Massachusetts Appointed to Consider the Expediency of Modifying the Laws Relating to the Registration of Births, Marriages, and Deaths, Presented March 3, 1849*, Mass. *House Document No. 65* (March 3, 1849), 3–54.

27. *Report of a General Plan for the Promotion of Public and Personal Health, Devised, Prepared and Recommended by the Commissioners Appointed Under a Resolve of the Legislature of Massachusetts, Relating to a Sanitary Survey of the State. Presented April 25, 1850* (Boston, 1850), 10, 201–5, 307–21, et passim.

28. EJ, "Autobiography," 188–89, HLHU; EJ to John C. Warren, November 21, 1849, Warren Papers, MHS; John C. Warren to EJ, October 9, December 15, 1849, EJ Papers, CLMHMS; *Report of a General Plan for the Promotion of Public and Personal Health*, 352–58. In his report Shattuck quoted with obvious approval Jarvis's remarks on prevention from his address before the Massachusetts Medical Society in 1849. See *Report of a General Plan for the Promotion of Public and Personal Health*, 11, 177, 247.

29. EJ, "Report of the Sanitary Commission of Massachusetts," *Boston Medical and Surgical Journal*, XLIV (March 5, 1851), 89–97.

30. EJ, "Report of the Sanitary Commission of Massachusetts," *American Journal of the Medical Sciences*, XXI (April 1851), 391–409.

31. EJ, "Houses & People. Concord Mass. 1810–1820," 249, mss. vol., CFPL.

32. EJ, "Autobiography," 189, HLHU.

33. Cf. Charles E. Rosenberg, *The Cholera Years: The United States in 1832, 1849, and 1866* (Chicago, 1962), 133–50.

34. *Report of a General Plan for the Promotion of Public and Personal Health*, 205–6.

35. EJ, "Treatises on Ventilation," *American Journal of the Medical Sciences*, XVIII (July 1849), 142, 147.

36. For an informative discussion of the ideology of statistics see

Philip Abrams, *The Origins of British Sociology: 1834-1914* (Chicago,1968), 3-30.

37. Cf. EJ, "Plan of a course of lectures," included with a letter from EJ to B.E. Cotting, July 29, 1854, EJLB, CLMHMS. For other divergencies of opinion within the ranks of sanitarians see Charles E. and Carroll S. Rosenberg, "Pietism and the Origins of the American Public Health Movement: A Note on John H. Griscom and Robert M. Hartley," *Journal of the History of Medicine and Allied Sciences,* XXIII (January 1968), 16-35.

38. EJ, "Sanitary Condition of Massachusetts and New England," American Medical Association, *Transactions,* III (1850), 247-66.

39. When the Massachusetts Medical Society petitioned for a General Board of Health in 1853, a joint legislative committee conceded that such an agency might "do much good in pointing out and perhaps correcting many evils which are now diminishing the value of human life among us." Nevertheless, it declined to endorse the proposal, preferring instead to support strengthened registration procedures (Mass. *House Document No. 50* [March 4, 1853], 2-3).

40. Rosenkrantz, *Public Health and the State,* 34-36.

41. Edward H. Barton to EJ, October 1, 1853, EJ Papers, CLMHMS; Robert C. Davis, "Social Research in America before the Civil War," *Journal of the History of the Behavioral Sciences,* VIII (January 1972), 69-85.

42. EJ, "Births, Marriages, and Deaths in Massachusetts," *American Journal of the Medical Sciences,* XXIV (July 1852), 147-64 (quote from p. 164).

43. Jarvis's correspondence on exchanges was voluminous. For examples see the following: John H. Griscom to EJ, August 18, 1848, May 9, July 11, 1853, June 10, 1854, March 3, 1864, September 16, 1867, T. Romenyn Beck to EJ, June 1, 24, September 9, 1852, January 3, May 4, June 8, October 20, November 8, 1853, G. Varrentrepp to EJ, August 9, 1872, March 9, 1873, EJ Papers, CLMHMS; EJ to T. Romenyn Beck, March 14, 1850, June 4, 1855, EJ to William Farr, June 10, 1850, EJ to T. Southwood Smith, June 10, 1850, EJ to Edward Cheshire, December 29, 1853, May 5, 1854, EJ to George Graham, June 10, 1853, April 25, 1854, November 1, 1855, August 24, 1857, EJ to Adolphe Quetelet, October 8, 1853, EJ to Charles Sumner, March 11, 1854, February 15, 1868, EJ to John P. Hale, October 25, 1865, EJ to William C. Waddell, November 2, 1866, EJ to Joseph Henry, May 27, 1861, April 8, August 17, 1866, June 24, October 26, 1869, EJ to A. Legoyt, November 16, 1860, July 17, 1865, July 2, 1870, EJLB, CLMHMS; EJ to Adolphe Quetelet, June 2, 1866,

Correspondence of A. Quetelet, Academie Royale de Belgique, Brussels, Belgium; EJ to Joseph Henry, January 16, 1863, March 5, 1866, July 27, October 26, 1869, October 25, 1870, December 24, 1872, Joseph Henry Papers, Smithsonian Institution, Washington, D.C.; A. Legoyt to EJ, August 30, 1871, G. Varrentrepp to EJ, March 7, 1874, May 8, 1876, EJ Papers, CFPL.

CHAPTER 5

1. For some critical comments about American society see EJ to Charles Sumner, September 21, 1845, Sumner Papers, HLHU.

2. *Report Made to the Legislature of Massachusetts, Upon Idiocy,* Mass. *Senate Document No. 51* (February 26, 1848), passim; *On the Causes of Idiocy; Being the Supplement to a Report by Dr. S. G. Howe . . . February 26, 1848* (Edinburgh, 1858), 2–3; Harold Schwartz, *Samuel Gridley Howe: Social Reformer 1801–1876* (Cambridge, 1956), 137–44.

3. See Isaac Hays to EJ, November 29, 1848, March 7, 1849, EJ Papers, CLMHMS. See also EJ to Samuel Gridley Howe, January 19, 1849, Howe Papers, HLHU.

4. EJ, "Reports on Idiocy," *American Journal of the Medical Sciences,* n.s. XVII (April 1849), 421–41. Jarvis's article drew the attention of Forbes Winslow, the eminent British psychiatrist, who immediately reprinted it in his own journal under the title "Causes, Cure, and Prevention of Idiocy," *Journal of Psychological Medicine and Mental Pathology,* III (July 1, 1850), 292–322. Howe also reprinted it in the Massachusetts School for the Idiotic and Feeble-Minded, *Annual Report,* XXVIII (1875), 77–105.

5. Hervey B. Wilbur to EJ, May 10, 1867, EJ Papers, CLMHMS.

6. For Jarvis's role in the school, see the following sources: EJ to Edward Hale, July 7, 1850, EJ to Daniel Whiting, July 7, 1850, EJ to Nathaniel Morton, August 17, 1850, EJ to A. Woodward, August 20, 1850, EJ to Nicholas Tillinghast, August 30, 1850, EJ to Samuel Gridley Howe, September 16, 1851, June 25, 1853, February 27, 1854, August 25, 1855, EJ to Mary A. Horton, November 16, 1863, EJ to O. Myrick, November 28, 1863, EJ to William A. Gordon, December 2, 1863, EJ to Samuel D. Wadsworth, July 8, 1867, EJ to Sarah M. Taylor, July 8, 1867, EJ to Andrew McFarland, September 13, 1867, Walter E. Fernald State School, Waverly, Mass.; EJ to Howe, February 27, 1854, EJ to George B. Emerson, February 27, 1854, EJ to Benjamin B. Scisson, January 12, 1855, EJLB, CLMHMS; EJ to Howe,

April 17, August 10, 1854, November 20, 1858, Howe Papers, HLHU; Howe to EJ, May 11, 1855, January 4, 30, March 8, 1858, February 3, 1859, September 6, 1860, February 27, 1867, April 8, 27, May 1, 1868, January 13, 1871, February 3, 1872, Isaac N. Kerlin to EJ, February 7, 1868, EJ Papers, CLMHMS; EJ to Francis W. Bird, October 2, 1858, Bird Papers, CLMHMS; Massachusetts School for Idiotic and Feeble-Minded Youth, *Annual Report*, IX (1856), 3-6, 23-26; ibid., XVI (1863), 20-21; ibid., XX (1867), 4-23; ibid., XXIII (1875), 45; ibid., XXIX (1876), 19-20; ibid., XXXVII (1884), 8-10; Mass. *Senate Document No. 25* (January 1861), 1-5.

7. Perkins Institution and Massachusetts Asylum for the Blind, *Annual Report*, XXXVI (1867), 9. This report was written by Jarvis.

8. EJ to David Cannon, July 19, August 12, 1850, EJ to John Shaw, October 17, 1850, Walter E. Fernald State School, Waverly, Mass.; Perkins Institution and Massachusetts Asylum for the Blind, *Annual Report*, XXXVI (1867), 12-14.

9. EJ, "The Influence of Distance from and Proximity to an Insane Hospital, on its Use by any People," *Boston Medical and Surgical Journal*, XLII (April 17, 1850), 209-22. Jarvis's methodology in this article was relatively crude; the use of counties as a category did not necessarily coincide with distance to a hospital.

10. Ohio Lunatic Asylum, *Annual Report*, VIII (1846), 34; ibid., X (1848), 44; ibid., XI (1849), 46-47; Maine Insane Hospital, *Annual Report*, X (1850), 36-37; D. Tilden Brown to EJ, April 20, 1855, EJ Papers, CLMHMS; EJ, "The Influence of Distance from, and Proximity to, an Insane Hospital, on its Use by any People," *American Journal of Insanity*, VII (January 1851), 281-85. Jarvis's concern with the placement of hospitals never abated. In 1866 he published a longer and updated version of the earlier article. His basic conclusion remained unchanged; use and distance were inversely related. See EJ, "Influence of Distance from and Nearness to an Insane Hospital on its Use by the People," *American Journal of Insanity*, XXII (January 1866), 361-406.

11. There are innumerable pamphlets and books dealing with this episode. The most recent is Robert Sullivan's *The Disappearance of Dr. Parkman* (Boston, 1971). For a defense of Shaw see Leonard W. Levy, *The Law of the Commonwealth and Chief Justice Shaw* (Cambridge, 1957), 218-28.

12. EJ to Luther V. Bell, July 3, 1850, EJLB, CLMHMS.

13. Boston *Daily Advertiser*, July 8, 9, 1850; EJ to Samuel Parkman, July 10, 1850, EJLB, CLMHMS.

14. EJ to the Committee of the Honorable Council, July 18, 1850,

Massachusetts Archives, Secretary of State's Office, State House, Boston, Mass.

15. Sullivan, *Disappearance of Dr. Parkman,* 201-2.

16. When the Association of Medical Superintendents of American Institutions for the Insane was in the process of being founded in 1844, Jarvis expressed the hope that the new organization would promote statistical studies of insanity. Conclusions based on the observations of a single individual could easily lead to false inferences; hence the experiences of "all the observors in the country" were necessary to determine "the true causes of insanity, and the real influences that remove it" (EJ to Samuel B. Woodward, October 12, 1844, Woodward Papers, AAS). See also Woodward to EJ, September 14, 1844, EJ Papers, CLMHMS, and the *American Journal of Insanity,* VI (July 1849), 59-60.

17. EJ, "On the Comparative Liability of Males and Females to Insanity, and Their Comparative Curability and Mortality When Insane," *American Journal of Insanity,* VII (October 1850), 142-71. This problem continued to interest Jarvis. See EJ to Thomas S. Kirkbride, March 13, 1857, Kirkbride Papers, IPH; EJ to Pliny Earle, June 29, August ?, 1857, Earle Papers, AAS; EJ to Samuel Gaskell, August 25, 1857, EJ to Kirkbride, April 2, 1859, EJ Papers, CLMHMS. For a general discussion of sex roles and medical thought see Charles E. Rosenberg, *No Other Gods: On Science and American Social Thought* (Baltimore, 1976), chaps. 2-3.

18. Cf. George Rosen, "Social Stress and Mental Disease from the Eighteenth Century to the Present: Some Origins of Social Psychiatry," *Milbank Memorial Fund Quarterly,* XXXVII (January 1959), 5-32. Given the role that psychiatrists defined for themselves, their predilection to identify civilization with mental disease was understandable. See Gerald N. Grob, *Mental Institutions in America: Social Policy to 1875* (New York, 1973), chap. 4.

19. EJ, "On the Supposed Increase of Insanity," *American Journal of Insanity,* VIII (April 1852), 333-64. A modified version was published under the title "Causes of Insanity," *Boston Medical and Surgical Journal,* XLV (November 12, 1851), 289-305, and circulated in pamphlet form *On the Causes of Insanity* (n.p., n.d.).

20. Boston *Daily Journal,* March 12, 1849; EJ, "Plan and Structure of Insane Hospitals," *Boston Medical and Surgical Journal,* XLIV (July 23, 1851), 494-97; *American Journal of Insanity,* IX (July 1852), 70; ibid., X (July 1853), 78; ibid., XI (July 1854), 48-49; EJ to Joel Parker, August 11, 1853, EJLB, CLMHMS.

21. Gerald N. Grob, *The State and the Mentally Ill: A History of*

Worcester State Hospital in Massachusetts 1830-1920 (Chapel Hill, 1966), chaps. 2–3.

22. Mass. *Senate Document No. 60* (March 9, 1854); Mass. *Senate Document No. 83* (March 1854); chap. 64, Resolve of April 24, 1854, in *Acts and Resolves Passed by the General Court of Massachusetts, in the Year 1854* (Boston, 1854), 438.

23. EJ, "Autobiography," 153, mss., HLHU; *Report on Insanity and Idiocy in Massachusetts, by the Commission on Lunacy, Under Resolve of the Legislature of 1854,* Mass. *House Document No. 144* (March 1, 1855), 189.

24. For eight months Jarvis devoted himself exclusively to this project, often working twelve to fourteen hours per day; he received $5 per day compensation from the state. See EJ, "Autobiography," 165, HLHU.

25. All of the manuscript returns can be found in the "Report of the Physicians of Massachusetts. Superintendents of Hospitals . . . and Others Describing the Insane and Idiotic Persons in the State of Massachusetts in 1855. Made to the Commissioners on Lunacy," mss. vol., CLMHMS. See also the *Report on Insanity and Idiocy in Massachusetts,* 11–16; *Medical Communications of the Massachusetts Medical Society,* 2d ser. V (Boston, 1860), 3–4; and EJ, "To the Medical Profession of Massachusetts," *Boston Medical and Surgical Journal,* LIII (November 22, 1855), 337–42.

26. George Brill to EJ, August 18, 1854, John Ware to EJ, September 30, 1854, Silas Brown to EJ, October 23, 1854, Charles M. Weeks to EJ, September 4, 1854, in "Report of the Physicians of Massachusetts. Superintendents of Hospitals . . . and Others Describing the Insane and Idiotic Persons in the State of Massachusetts in 1855. Made to the Commissioners on Lunacy," CLMHMS.

27. E.B. Moore to EJ, August 21, 1854, ibid.

28. *Report on Insanity and Idiocy in Massachusetts,* 17–18.

29. Ibid., 45, 52–56.

30. Ibid., 59–62.

31. Ibid., 62–63, 112. In his published report Jarvis did not provide data on length of institutionalization or duration of illness. While the manuscript census returns provided some information on this subject, their accuracy insofar as immigrants were concerned was of dubious reliability. Under these circumstances Jarvis's own attitudes became the most important determinant of his explanation.

The responses of the superintendents to Jarvis's questionnaire also pose an interesting historical problem. In general, psychiatrists tended to make the same distinctions between the native and immigrant insane as Jarvis. On the other hand, their contacts with *individual* patients may not have completely reflected the general stereotype to which they subscribed—a not uncommon phenomenon.

32. For Jarvis's identification of social problems with immigration see EJ to A. Quetelet, October 8, 1853, EJ to Louis Dwight, November ?, 1853, EJ to Edwin Chadwick, June 10, 1853, EJLB, CLMHMS.

33. Cf. Barbara M. Solomon, *Ancestors and Immigrants: A Changing New England Tradition* (Cambridge, 1956), on the declining democratic faith of the Brahmin intelligentsia.

34. *Report on Insanity and Idiocy in Massachusetts,* 65–68.

35. Ibid., 104–33.

36. Ibid., 134–35. Some copies of these letters are preserved in the EJLB, CLMHMS.

37. The recommendations of the Association of Medical Superintendents of American Institutions for the Insane can be found in the *American Journal of Insanity,* VIII (July 1851), 79–81.

38. *Report on Insanity and Idiocy in Massachusetts,* 135–43.

39. Ibid., 143–45.

40. Ibid., 145–47.

41. Ibid., 147–54.

42. Ibid., 184.

43. EJ, "Autobiography," 162–64, HLHU; EJ, "To the Medical Profession of Massachusetts," *Boston Medical and Surgical Journal,* LIII (November 22, 1855), 337–42; ibid., LIII (December 20, 1855), 433; Mass. *House Document No. 282* (April 26, 1855); chap. 454, Act of May 21, 1855, in *Acts and Resolves Passed by the General Court of Massachusetts, in the Year 1855* (Boston, 1855), 870; EJ to Pliny Earle, April 29, 1857, Earle Papers, AAS.

Jarvis himself noted that he had not dealt in detail with the problems presented by idiocy, since the legislature's mandate was largely phrased in terms of the mentally ill. Consequently, he simply gathered some raw data on idiocy in the hope that it would serve in the future as a basis for developing a humane and comprehensive policy on idiocy. See the *Report on Insanity and Idiocy in Massachusetts,* 79.

44. EJ, *Address Delivered at the Laying of the Corner Stone of the Insane Hospital, at Northampton, Massachusetts* (Northampton, 1856). In this address Jarvis spelled out his views on insanity and the proper contours of public policy.

45. EJ to Thomas S. Kirkbride, July 21, 1855, Kirkbride Papers, IPH; EJ to William Bridgman, July 27, 1855, EJ to Samuel Stanley, March 26, June 14, 1856, EJ to George Chandler, April 12, 1856, EJ to George C.S. Choate, April 12, 1856, EJLB, CLMHMS; Howe to EJ, Feb-

ruary 11, 1856, Luther V. Bell to EJ, January 11, March 22, June 2, 25, 1856, February 12, 1858, EJ Papers, CLMHMS; Mass. *House Document No. 18* (January 9, 1856), 2–3; ibid., *No. 138* (March 25, 1856), 1–4; ibid., *No. 215* (April 22, 1856); ibid., *No. 146* (March 16, 1858), 1–8; *Boston Medical and Surgical Journal,* LIV (April 24, 1856), 246.

46. Benjamin Barrett to EJ, December 28, 1856, February 6, April 28, July 11, 1857, EJ Papers, CLMHMS; EJ to Barrett, April 14, January (?) 30, 1857, EJ to Josiah Bartlett, April 14, 1857, EJLB, CLMHMS.

47. EJ, "Autobiography," 165, HLHU.

48. Cf. David J. Rothman, *The Discovery of the Asylum: Social Order and Disorder in the New Republic* (Boston, 1971), and Christopher Lasch, "Origins of the Asylum," in his collection of essays entitled *The World of Nations: Reflections on American History, Politics, and Culture* (New York, 1973), 3–17.

49. EJ to Pliny Earle, April 29, 1857, Earle Papers, AAS; EJ to James Deane, September 25, 1855, EJ to George S. Willis, September 25, 1855, EJ to Levi Lincoln, September 27, 1855, EJ to James Nye, September 28, 1855, EJ to George H. Babbit, October 4, 1855, EJ to R.W.S. Lutwidge, November 13, 1855, EJ to Joseph Henry, May 16, 1857, EJLB, CLMHMS; D. Tilden Brown to EJ, April 20, 1855, John S. Butler to EJ, May 12, 1855, D.H. Trezevant to EJ, November 28, 1855, Thomas R. Elliott to EJ, February 11, 1856, Samuel P. Hildreth to EJ, February 18, 1856, J.C. Rutherford to EJ, April 22, 1856, R.C. Hopkins to EJ, December 27, 1856, James Coxe to EJ, June 4, 1857, EJ Papers, CLMHMS; *American Journal of Insanity,* XII (July 1855), 94–97.

50. *Boston Medical and Surgical Journal,* LIII (December 20, 1855), 433; "The Massachusetts Lunacy Commission," *American Journal of Insanity,* XII (January 1856), 259–66; T.R. Beck, "Insanity and Idiocy in Massachusetts," *American Journal of Insanity,* XII (October 1855), 146–82.

51. Earle's review appeared in the *American Journal of the Medical Sciences,* n.s. XXXI (April 1856), 429–36.

52. *Journal of Prison Discipline and Philanthropy,* XI (January 1856), 10–24.

53. See Ray's *A Treatise on the Medical Jurisprudence of Insanity* (Boston, 1838). This book went through four subsequent editions and remained a classic. Ray originally preferred Howe as the reviewer of Jarvis's report. See Isaac Ray to EJ, June 16, November 3, 1855, EJ Papers, CLMHMS.

54. Curiously enough, Ray (and most others) disregarded the fig-

ures listing the number of insane residents of Massachusetts in hospitals by sex, nativity, and prognosis, which did not support the allegation that the native insane had higher curability rates than immigrants. See the *Report on Insanity and Idiocy in Massachusetts,* 112.

55. Isaac Ray, "Statistics of Insanity in Massachusetts," *North American Review,* LXXXII (January 1856), 78–100. By the 1860s Ray had reversed his approval of separate institutions for incurable patients. See Ray to Dorothea L. Dix, December 29, 1869, Dix Papers, HLHU.

In the psychiatric literature of the 1850s and 1860s the *Report on Insanity* was often held up as a model. The annual reports of American mental hospitals during these decades abound with references. See also J.A. Reed to EJ, September 6, 1863, Samuel D. Hastings to EJ, November 1, 1867, Henry P. Bowditch to EJ, March 10, 1875, EJ Papers, CLMHMS, and Isaac Ray, *Address Delivered by Isaac Ray, M.D., of Philadelphia, on the Occasion of Laying the Corner Stone of the State Hospital for the Insane, at Danville, Pa. August 26, 1869* (Harrisburg, 1869), 17.

56. Compare Jarvis's statement about the Irish in his letter to the Earl of Carlisle, November 1, 1855, EJLB, CLMHMS, with the statement in the *Boston Medical and Surgical Journal,* XLV (January 28, 1852), 537. See also Grob, *State and the Mentally Ill,* chap. 5.

57. *American Journal of Insanity,* XIII (July 1856), 83; EJ, "Criminal Insane. Insane Transgressors and Insane Convicts," ibid., XIII (January 1857), 195–231. See also EJ to E.K. Hunt, January 14, 1856, EJLB, CLMHMS.

58. EJ to Horace A. Buttolph, May 5, 1854, William Jones Rhees Collection, Henry E. Huntington Library, San Marino, California; EJ to Henry Barnard, February 8, 1858, EJLB, CLMHMS; *American Journal of Insanity,* XI (July 1854), 48; EJ, "Tendency of Misdirected Education and the Unbalanced Mind to Produce Insanity," *American Journal of Education,* IV (March 1858), 591–612, reprinted in the British periodical *Journal of Psychological Medicine and Mental Pathology,* XI (July 1, 1858), 424–44.

59. EJ, "Causes of Mental Disease," *North American Review,* LXXXIX (October 1859), 316–39.

CHAPTER 6

1. EJ to Louis Dwight, November ?, 1853, EJLB, CLMHMS.
2. This discussion of Quetelet is based on Victor L. Hilts, "Statis-

tics and Social Science," in *Foundations of Scientific Method: The Nineteenth Century*, ed. Ronald N. Giere and Richard S. Westfall (Bloomington, 1973), 206–33, and Frank H. Hankins, *Adolphe Quetelet as Statistician* (New York, 1908).

3. EJ to A. Quetelet, October 8, 1853, EJLB, CLMHMS.

4. Jarvis's desire for comparative materials was evident in his communication to the London Statistical Society. "I am desirous to obtain every thing relative to population & humanity, to the general health, cultivation & progress of civilization, also to the depressions—insanity —other sickness, poverty & crime, in Europe, & am glad to make such returns, such as I have sent to & through you." EJ to Edward Cheshire, November 13, 1855, EJLB, CLMHMS.

5. See the "Report of the Secretary of the Treasury," 28th Cong., 2d session, *Senate Document No. 21* (January 6, 1845), 2–4, and "Letters Addressed to the Hon. John Davis, Concerning the Census of 1849, by Nahum Capen and Jesse Chickering," 30th Cong., 2d session, *Senate Miscellaneous Document No. 64* (March 3, 1849), 26.

6. "Records of the American Statistical Association 1839–1872," mss. vol., 35–38, 41–43, ASA; EJ to William Damrell, December 26, 1857, EJ to J.D.B. De Bow, July 10, 1853, EJLB, CLMHMS; *Statistical View of the United States . . . Being a Compendium of the Seventh Census* (Washington, D.C., 1854), 12ff; EJ, "Autobiography," 216, mss., HLHU; Robert C. Davis, "Social Research in America before the Civil War," *Journal of the History of the Behavioral Sciences,* VIII (January 1972), 75–77; Carroll D. Wright and William C. Hunt, *The History and Growth of the United States Census* (Washington, D.C., 1900), 39ff. Unfortunately, Jarvis's original letter to Kennedy in 1849 does not seem to have survived. For biographical data on Kennedy see the Kennedy folder, Walter Willcox Papers, LC.

7. EJ, "Autobiography," 217, HLHU; "Report of the Superintendent of the Census," 32d Cong., 1st session, *House Executive Document No. 2* (December 2, 1851), 222.

8. For Jarvis's continuing interest in the census during this period see Edward H. Barton to EJ, September 18, 1852, March 16, 1854, Stephen W. Williams to EJ, July 12, 19, 1852, EJ Papers, CLMHMS; *Medical Communications of the Massachusetts Medical Society,* 2d ser. VIII (Boston, 1854), 78; 33d Cong., 1st session, *Senate Executive Document No. 9* (December 20, 1853), 6–7.

9. For De Bow's career see Ottis C. Skipper, *J.D.B. De Bow: Magazinist of the Old South* (Athens, Ga., 1958), and the De Bow Papers, Perkins Library, Duke University, Durham, North Carolina.

10. EJ to De Bow, July 10, 1853, EJLB, CLMHMS. For some discussion

of the preliminary returns for Maryland see 32d Cong., 1st session, *Senate Report No. 276* (June 28, 1852).

11. EJ to De Bow, August 30, 1853, EJLB, CLMHMS.

12. Jesse Chickering, *Immigration into the United States* (Boston, 1848), 25, 58–66, et passim. The basic difficulty of determining the number of immigrants and their descendants grew out of the fact that neither the sixth nor the seventh census provided the requisite data. Both of these censuses gathered statistics on native and foreign born; consequently, children of the latter were listed in the former category.

13. Jarvis was especially critical of the fact that an abstract of the census published in early 1853 included Kennedy's report for 1851 without an explicit repudiation of its fallacious reasoning. Kennedy had taken the number of foreigners arriving between 1790 and 1810 together with those arriving in each of the decades between 1810 and 1850, and estimated their natural increase. Such a procedure, noted Jarvis, had fundamental flaws, for it assumed that no foreigners (or their children) migrating to the United States in the sixty years preceding 1850 had ever died. Nor could mortality tables be applied easily as a corrective, for there was no record of the ages of immigrants (with the exception of the single year of 1847). The use of existing mortality tables was further limited by the fact that immigrants had far higher mortality rates than natives. Kennedy's report for 1852, on the other hand, was a distinct improvement because it applied the law of mortality to the foreign-born. Nevertheless, Jarvis felt that a deduction of 10 percent from the expectation of life for immigrants was simply too small; Kennedy still overestimated the number of foreign-born and their descendants. EJ to De Bow, September 20, 26, 28, 1853, EJLB, CLMHMS. Jarvis was referring to Kennedy's estimates in *The Seventh Census. Report of the Superintendent of the Census for December 1, 1852; to which is Appended the Report for December 1, 1851* (Washington, D.C., 1853), 14–15, 118–20, 132–33 (this source was more popularly known as the *Abstract of the Seventh Census,* the title that appeared on the cover of the volume). The figures for 1847 appeared in "Passengers Arriving in the United States," 30th Cong., 1st session, *House Executive Document No. 47* (March 3, 1848).

14. EJ to De Bow, September 20, 23, 1853, EJLB, CLMHMS.

15. *The Seventh Census of the United States: 1850* (Washington, D.C., 1853); EJ to De Bow, January 18, 21, 30, 1854, EJLB, CLMHMS.

16. EJ to De Bow, February 15, 1854, EJLB, CLMHMS; *The Seventh Census. Report of the Superintendent of the Census for December 1, 1852; to which is Appended the Report for December 1, 1851,* 28;

New York *Herald,* February 9, 1854. See also EJ to Charles Sumner, April 15, 1854, EJLB, CLMHMS.

17. EJ to De Bow, February 15, March 20, 1854, EJLB, CLMHMS.

18. J.D.B. De Bow, *Statistical View of the United States . . . Being a Compendium of the Seventh Census* (Washington, D.C., 1854), 113, 120–22, 161–64. See also EJ to De Bow, July 17, November 29, 1854, EJLB, CLMHMS.

19. *Mortality Statistics of the Seventh Census of the United States, 1850* (Washington, D.C., 1855), 33rd Cong., 2d session, *House Executive Document No. 98* (1855), 2; Skipper, *J.D.B. De Bow,* 77–78.

20. EJ to De Bow, August 30, September 20, 1853, March 13, 1854, January 19, 1856, EJLB, CLMHMS.

21. EJ to De Bow, February 15, August 24, September 18, 1855, ibid. De Bow reprinted in a slightly different version Jarvis's letter of September 18 (in printed form it was dated September 22) in the *Mortality Statistics of the Seventh Census,* 45–48.

22. *Mortality Statistics of the Seventh Census,* 8–11.

23. EJ to De Bow, January 19, 1856, EJLB, CLMHMS.

24. Cf. Jarvis's angry reaction upon learning of remarks in Congress relating to longevity, particularly of free and slave blacks. EJ to Charles Sumner, April 15, 1854, EJLB, CLMHMS.

25. EJ to De Bow, September 22, November 17, 1855, January 19, April 19, May 30, 1856, EJ to William S. Damrell, June 14, December 3, 1856, December 26, 1857, ibid.

26. EJ to De Bow, April 19, May 30, 1856, February 21, November 5, December 26, 1857, November 29, 1858, EJ to Charles Sumner, April 19, 1856, EJ to William S. Damrell, June 14, December 3, 1856, February 19, December 26, 1857, EJ to Henry Wilson, November 11, 1857, EJ to James Dixon, January 1, 1858, EJ to Charles Francis Adams, October 31, 1859, February 20, 1860, EJ to J.C.G. Kennedy, February 20, 1860, EJ to James Wynne, November 16, 1860, EJ to Oakes Ames, November 10, 1863, ibid.; EJ to Charles Sumner, December 26, 1859, Sumner Papers, HLHU; 36th Cong., 1st session, *House Report No. 91* (March 19, 1860); 36th Cong., 1st session, *Congressional Globe,* 1232, 1603–5.

27. EJ to James Harlan, September 5, 1865, August 18, 1866, EJ to William B. Washburn, June 19, 1866, January 18, December 7, 1867, EJ to Henry Wilson, June 22, December 14, 1866, December 13, 1867, EJ to John W. Forney, August 6, 1866, EJ to James S. Wilson, August 13, 27, 1866, EJ to Henry B. Anthony, September 6, December 12, 1866, EJ to Charles Sumner, December 6, 14, 1866, Janu-

ary 15, December 13, 18, 31, 1867, June 10, 1868, December 30, 1869, EJ to Timothy O. Howe, December 14, 17, 1866, January 1, 1868, EJ to G. Twichell, November 12, 1867, EJ to George S. Boutwell, December 5, 1867, December 2, 1873, April 1, 1874, EJ to Nathaniel Banks, December 10, 1867, EJ to Thomas D. Eliot, December 10, 1867, EJ to Justin Morrill, December 31, 1867, June 10, 1868, EJ to James A. Garfield, November ?, 1869, EJ to William A. Richardson, May 6, 1874, EJLB, CLMHMS; EJ to James A. Garfield, March 16, 1870, Garfield Papers, LC; Charles Sumner to EJ, June 16, 1868, Robert W. Wood to EJ, December 13, 18, 1867, EJ Papers, CLMHMS; 39th Cong., 1st session, *Congressional Globe,* 3373–74, 3382, 3397; 39th Cong., 1st session, *House Journal,* 798, 891–92, and *Senate Journal,* 370–71; 40th Cong., 1st session, *Senate Journal,* 55; 40th Cong., 2d session, *House Journal,* 58; 43d Cong., 1st session, *Congressional Record,* 140, 631; 43d Cong., 1st session, *Senate Journal,* 60, 143, 195, 236, 335, 347, 370, and *House Journal,* 423, 480, 574–75, 591, 656; 43d Cong., 1st session, *Senate Report No. 13* (January 14, 1874).

28. EJ to Charles Sumner, June 24, 1853, EJLB, CLMHMS. See also EJ to Edwin Chadwick, June 10, 1853, ibid.

29. EJ, "Registration of Births, Marriages, and Deaths," *American Journal of the Medical Sciences,* XXIX (April 1855), 407–30; EJ to Isaac Hays, January 21, 1854, EJLB, CLMHMS.

30. EJ, "Report on Registration of Births, Marriages, and Deaths," American Medical Association, *Transactions,* XI (1858), 525–47; Edwin M. Snow to EJ, October 12, 1858, January 7, 1861, EJ Papers, CLMHMS; "Records of the American Statistical Association 1839–1872," 63, ASA; Benjamin Cutter to EJ, October 21, 1857, January 20, 1858, May 20, 1859, EJ Papers, CLMHMS; Mass. *Senate Document No. 46* (March 9, 1858), *Senate Document No. 111* (March 15, 1859).

31. James Wynne, *Report on the Vital Statistics of the United States, Made to the Mutual Life Insurance Company of New York* (New York, 1857); Shepard B. Clough, *A Century of American Life Insurance: A History of the Mutual Life Insurance Company of New York 1843–1943* (New York, 1946), 81.

32. EJ to Isaac Hays, January 31, 1859, EJLB, CLMHMS.

33. Jarvis's review of Wynne's book appeared in the *American Journal of the Medical Sciences,* XXVII (April 1859), 458–86.

34. EJ to Rev. Henry W. Bellows, November 2, 1857, Bellows Papers, MHS.

35. EJ to Rev. Louis Dwight, November ?, 1853, EJLB, CLMHMS.

36. EJ to Henry W. Bellows, November 2, 1857, Bellows Papers,

MHS. Jarvis repeated these findings in his paper in London at the International Statistical Congress in 1860. See EJ, "Comparative Liability of Males and Females to Various Kinds of Crime," *Report of the Proceedings of the Fourth Session of the International Statistical Congress, Held in London July 16th, 1860, and the Five Following Days* (London, 1861), 446–47. In his letter to Dwight in 1853 Jarvis offered a comprehensive program for the collection of crime statistics. He suggested the adoption of a uniform system of reporting on criminals giving the following information: (1) number committed to prison by year, broken down by county (including total population), county of birth, race, and sex; (2) foreign born (including their population by county); (3) classes of crime, nativity, and sex; (4) identical with preceding table, but aggregated for a number of years; (5) age, sex, and place where crime was committed; (6) identical with preceding table, but aggregated for a number of years; (7) level of education, class of crime, and nativity; (8) recidivist rate, nativity, and sex; (9) identical with preceding table, but aggregated for a number of years. EJ to Louis Dwight, November ?, 1853, EJLB, CLMHMS.

37. *Rules and Regulations of the Board of Health, of the Town of Dorchester, Massachusetts. Adopted, August 15th, 1855* (Dorchester, 1855); EJ, "Autobiography," 194, HLHU; EJ to George H. Snelling, March 30, 1857, April 2, 1859, in Mass. *Senate Document No. 186* (April 1859), 10–15.

CHAPTER 7

1. Samuel Gridley Howe to EJ, May 11, 1855, February 11, 1856, Luther V. Bell to EJ, January 14, 1859, EJ Papers, CLMHMS; EJ to Luther V. Bell, January 28, 1859, EJLB, CLMHMS.

2. EJ to Jacob Bigelow, May ?, 1860, EJ to Charles Hemenway, June 26, 1860, EJLB, CLMHMS; EJ, "Autobiography," 255, HLHU.

3. EJ to Almira Jarvis, March 8, 9, 13, 18, 21, 22, 1860, EJEL, CFPL.

4. EJ to Almira Jarvis, March 24, 25, 26, 28, 29, 31, April 2, 3, 4, 5, 6, 8, 9, 11, 12, 14, 15, 16, 18, 19, 21, 22, 1860, ibid.; EJ to Howe, June 1, 1860, Howe Papers, HLHU; EJ to Pliny Earle, December 1, 1860, Earle Papers, AAS.

5. EJ to Jacob Bigelow, May ?, 1860, EJLB, CLMHMS; EJ to Almira Jarvis, May 31, June 1, 1860, EJEL, CFPL.

6. EJ to Almira Jarvis, June 4, 7, 8, 9, 11, 12, 14, 17, 18, 22, 25, 28, 29, July 1, 3, 1860, EJEL, CFPL.

7. EJ to Almira Jarvis, July 8, 1860, ibid.

8. EJ to Almira Jarvis, July 12, 23, 1860, ibid.

9. "Records of the American Statistical Association 1839–1872," mss. vol., 72, ASA; Communication to EJ from the American Statistical Association, 1860, EJ Papers, CFPL; EJ to Almira Jarvis, July 15, ?, 1860, EJEL, CFPL; EJ to Augustus B. Longstreet, November 13, 1860, EJLB, CLMHMS. Jarvis later attempted to collect payment for his presence at the Congress, arguing that he was entitled to a portion of the funds appropriated by Congress for this purpose. See EJ to Longstreet, November 13, 1860, EJLB, CLMHMS.

10. *Report of the Proceedings of the Fourth Session of the International Statistical Congress, Held in London July 16th, 1860, and the Five Following Days* (London, 1861), 12; EJ to Almira Jarvis, July ?, 1860, EJEL, CFPL; Victor Ullman, *Martin R. Delany: The Beginnings of Black Nationalism* (Boston, 1971), 238ff.; Frank A. Rollin, *Life and Public Services of Martin R. Delany* (Boston, 1868), 99–133.

11. EJ to Almira Jarvis, July ?, 1860, EJEL, CFPL; Ullman, *Martin R. Delany*, 241–45.

12. *Report of the Proceedings of the Fourth Session of the International Statistical Congress*, 51–55, 176, 264–67, 271–72, 277–83, 446–47, 497–99. Just prior to the opening session of the congress, Jarvis delivered a paper describing the Massachusetts system of taxation before a meeting of the British Association for the Advancement of Science in Oxford. See EJ, "On the System of Taxation Prevailing in the United States, and Especially in Massachusetts," *Journal of the Statistical Society of London*, XXIII (September 1860), 370–78.

13. EJ to Almira Jarvis, July 18, 19, 22, 1860, EJEL, CFPL; EJ to William Farr, November 26, 1860, EJLB, CLMHMS.

14. EJ to Almira Jarvis, July 28, 31, August 1, 4, 5, 10, 11, 1860, EJEL, CFPL. For Jarvis's recollections of his trip see his "Autobiography," 255–321, HLHU.

15. EJ to Almira Jarvis, May 10, 23, 24, 1860, EJEL, CFPL.

16. Cf. Barbara M. Solomon, *Ancestors and Immigrants: A Changing New England Tradition* (Cambridge, 1956), passim.

17. EJ, "Autobiography," 198–99, 242–43, HLHU; *Boston Medical and Surgical Journal*, LXIII (January 24, 1861), 525–26; ibid., LXIV (February 14, 1861), 57; "Records of the American Statistical Association 1839–1872," 71½, ASA.

18. *Proceedings and Debates of the Fourth National Quarantine and Sanitary Convention, Held in the City of Boston, June 14, 15, and 16, 1860* (Boston, 1860), 123, 126; Barbara G. Rosenkrantz, *Public Health and the State: Changing Views in Massachusetts, 1842–1936* (Cambridge, 1972), 40.

19. *Memorial of the Boston Sanitary Association to the Legislature of Massachusetts, Asking for the Establishment of a Board of Health and of Vital Statistics* (Boston, 1861), 1–31, also in Mass. *House Document No. 112* (February 15, 1861).

20. EJ to Governor John A. Andrew, February 11, 1861, Andrew Papers, MHS; Josiah Curtis to EJ, February 5, March 5, 8, 21, April 13, 14, 1861, John Ware to EJ, December 13, 1861, January 14, 23, 1863, Lyman Bartlett to EJ, December 25, 1861, Charles Sewall to EJ, March 25, 1862, Horace Wakefield to EJ, January 2, February 2, 1863, EJ Papers, CLMHMS; EJ to Andrew, March 24, 1862, EJLB, CLMHMS; Mass. *Senate Document No. 127* (March 27, 1861); Governor's address, in *Acts and Resolves Passed by the General Court of Massachusetts, in the Year 1862* (Boston, 1862), 272; Mass. *Senate Document No. 82* (March 12, 1862); *Medical Communications of the Massachusetts Medical Society*, 2d ser. X (Boston, 1866), 67.

21. John L.S. Thompson to EJ, January 28, 1862, Josiah Bartlett to EJ, December 26, 1862, EJ Papers, CLMHMS; EJ, "Autobiography," 199–201, HLHU.

22. A few years earlier the Massachusetts Medical Society attempted to set up a system whereby all physicians would register the diseases of their patients. The project was a dismal failure; Dr. Benjamin Cutter reported that those with large practices could not comply and those with small practices would not. See Cutter to EJ, October 21, 1857, January 20, May 17, 1858, May 20, 1859, EJ Papers, CLMHMS.

23. Gerald N. Grob, *The State and the Mentally Ill: A History of Worcester State Hospital in Massachusetts, 1830-1920* (Chapel Hill, 1966), 180ff.

24. Samuel Gridley Howe to EJ, November 11, 1864 (1863?), EJ Papers, CLMHMS.

25. See Harold M. Hyman, *A More Perfect Union: The Impact of the Civil War and Reconstruction on the Constitution* (New York, 1973), Chap. XVIII.

26. Founded within weeks after the outbreak of war, the United States Sanitary Commission sought to apply the principles of public health to the nation's armed forces. Led by Henry W. Bellows (a prominent Unitarian minister), Dr. Elisha Harris (a leading sanitarian), and Frederick Law Olmsted (the famous commentator on the prewar South and a leading urban architect)—all from New York City —the new agency attempted to fuse "scientific" principles with modern organizational techniques. See William Q. Maxwell, *Lincoln's Fifth Wheel: The Political History of the United States Sanitary Commission* (New York, 1956). For a different interpretation consult

George M. Fredrickson, *The Inner Civil War: Northern Intellectuals and the Crisis of the Union* (New York, 1965), Chap. VII.

27. 37th Cong., 1st session, *Senate Miscellaneous Document No. 2* (July 12, 1861), 1–5.

28. EJ, "Sanitary Condition of the Army," *Atlantic Monthly*, X (October 1862), 463–97; EJ to George Nichols, August 18, September 17, 1862, Nichols Papers, HLHU. In preparing this article Jarvis relied on information from British colleagues. See EJ to John Sutherland, June 11, 1861, EJLB, CLMHMS; Ira Russell to EJ, December 4, 30, 1861, Josiah Curtis to EJ, December 15, 19, 1861, April 20, 1862, John Sutherland to EJ, March 15, 1863, EJ Papers, CLMHMS.

29. Ray to EJ, October 5, 1862, EJ Papers, CLMHMS.

30. EJ commissions as sanitary inspector, October 2, 1862, April 20, 1863, EJ Papers, CFPL; *Boston Medical and Surgical Journal*, LXVII (October 9, 1862), 207–8; ibid. (December 4, 1862), 363–67; ibid. (December 11, 1862), 381–84; ibid., LXVIII (April 9, 1863), 206; EJ to Elisha Harris, February 16, 1866, EJLB, CLMHMS.

31. EJ to W.H. Van Buren, October 20, 1862, EJLB, CLMHMS. The dispute between the sanitary commission and the Army's medical bureau grew out of differing concerns. The former was preoccupied with the preservation of health and the prevention of disease, the latter with the maintenance of the command authority that it deemed indispensable to military success.

32. EJ to Henry G. Clark, February 12, 1863, EJ to Charles A. Lee, June 26, 1865, EJ to Elisha Harris, February 16, 1866, ibid.; Edwin M. Snow to EJ, April 3, 1863, January 16, 1864, Samuel F. Haven to EJ, June 3, 1863, EJ Papers, CLMHMS; Henry G. Clark, *Department of the Special Inspection of the General Hospitals, U.S.A., Third (Preliminary) Report to the Committee, May, 1863* (New York, 1864), in *Documents of the U.S. Sanitary Commission*, No. 79; Maxwell, *Lincoln's Fifth Wheel*, 308. A search of the massive (but uncatalogued) United States Sanitary Commission Papers at the New York Public Library failed to uncover Jarvis's original report.

33. *American Journal of Insanity*, XIV (July 1857), 81–87, 89–90; EJ, "Distribution of Lunatic Hospital Reports," ibid., XIV (January 1858), 248–53; ibid., XV (July 1858), 120, 126–28. See also ibid., XIX (July 1862), 82–85, XXX (October 1873), 196.

34. EJ, "Law of Insanity, and Hospitals for the Insane in Massachusetts," *Monthly Law Reporter*, XXII (November 1859), 385–409; EJ to Judge Parker, November 19, 1859, EJLB, CLMHMS.

35. Chap. 73, *The General Statutes of the Commonwealth of Massachusetts* (Boston, 1860), 406–13. The only response to Jarvis's

article came from Ray, who maintained that Jarvis misunderstood the recommendation pertaining to a commission. Ray insisted that he had urged the establishment of temporary commissions whose authority was "limited to those few cases where the family do not wish to assume the responsibility" of commitment; the overwhelming majority of commitments would continue to be inaugurated by the family. Ray was probably overly sensitive, for Jarvis made it clear that he was proposing a sharply modified version of the commission concept. See Ray to EJ, January 20, 1860, EJ Papers, CLMHMS.

36. Mass. *House Document No. 57* (February 1862), 1–8; Governor's address, in *Acts and Resolves Passed by the General Court of Massachusetts, in the Year 1862* (Boston, 1862), 269–70; Gerald N. Grob, *Mental Institutions in America: Social Policy to 1875* (New York, 1973), 263ff.

37. Mass. *Senate Document No. 164* (April 21, 1862), 1–17; chap. 223, "An Act Concerning State Lunatic Hospitals and Insane and Idiotic Persons," in *Acts and Resolves Passed by the General Court of Massachusetts, in the Year 1862,* 193–97; EJ, "Autobiography," 169, HLHU.

In general, Jarvis rejected allegations that hospital superintendents or other physicians had unlimited authority to deprive insane persons of their personal liberty and often abused this power. When L. Clarke Davis launched an attack upon commitment procedures that mentioned Thomas S. Kirkbride in an unfavorable light, Jarvis immediately wrote to Kirkbride and offered support. See EJ to Kirkbride, May 28, 1868, Kirkbride Papers, IPH; L. Clarke Davis, "A Modern Lettre de Cachet," *Atlantic Monthly,* XXI (May 1868), 588–602. Isaac Ray was so incensed that he published a strong rejoinder to Davis entitled " 'A modern Lettre de Cachet' Reviewed," *Atlantic Monthly,* XXII (August 1868), 227–43.

38. Mass. *Senate Document No. 10* (January 1863), 1–2; Mass. *Senate Document No. 72* (February 23, 1864), 1–20; *Acts and Resolves Passed by the General Court of Massachusetts, in the Year 1863* (Boston, 1863), 587; chap. 288, *Acts and Resolves Passed by the General Court of Massachusetts, in the Year 1864* (Boston, 1864), 262–64.

39. EJ to Governor John A. Andrew, February 11, 1861, Andrew Papers, MHS.

40. Ibid. For the activities and attitude of this agency see *Report of the Commissioners of Alien Passengers and Foreign Paupers, 1859,* Mass. *Public Document No. 14* (1860), 10, and Grob, *The State and the Mentally Ill,* chap. 5.

41. Merrick Bemis to EJ, February 12, 1861, October 15, November 21, December 3, 12, 13, 16, 1862, January 19, March 16, October 4, November 20, 1863, April 11, 1864, January 5, 10, 1865, EJ Papers, CLMHMS; EJ to Bemis, December 1, 1862, EJ to William T. Merrifield, February 4, 1863, EJ to P. Emory Aldrich, November 30, 1863, EJLB, CLMHMS.

42. Worcester State Lunatic Hospital, *Annual Report*, XXX (1862), 11ff.

43. Ibid., 18ff.

44. Ibid., 29–47. See also EJ, "Mechanical and Other Employments for Patients in the British Lunatic Asylums," *American Journal of Insanity*, XIX (October 1862), 129–46.

45. Worcester State Lunatic Hospital, *Annual Report*, XXXI (1863), 3–36; EJ to Jacob H. Land, April 11, 1864 (2 letters), EJLB, CLMHMS; EJ to Pliny Earle, October 13, 28, December 26, 1864, February 10, 1865, Earle Papers, AAS.

46. Mass. *House Document No. 1* (January 1865), 1–27; Mass. Board of State Charities, *Annual Report*, I (1864), xiii–xviii; Grob, *The State and the Mentally Ill*, 206–7.

47. EJ, "Autobiography," 172–76, HLHU; Robert W. Hooper to EJ, February 6, 1866, EJ Papers, CLMHMS.

48. For a discussion of these issues see Grob, *Mental Institutions in America*, chaps. 7–8.

49. EJ, "On the Proper Functions of Private Institutions or Homes for the Insane," *American Journal of Insanity*, XVII (July 1860), 19–31.

50. Ibid., 35–43.

51. Ray to EJ, November 21, 1863, EJ Papers, CLMHMS. See also Ray's comments in Butler Hospital for the Insane, *Annual Report*, XVI (1862), 14–25.

52. EJ to Thomas S. Kirkbride, September 20, 1860, Kirkbride Papers, IPH. See also EJ to Samuel Gridley Howe, June 1, 1860, Howe Papers, HLHU, and EJ to Pliny Earle, December 1, 1860, Earle Papers, AAS.

53. EJ, "Mechanical and Other Employments for Patients in the British Lunatic Asylums," *American Journal of Insanity*, XIX (October 1862), 129–46.

54. Ibid., 54–71. See also Pliny Earle to EJ, December 8, 1860, Isaac Ray to EJ, September 29, 1860, EJ Papers, CLMHMS; Worcester State Lunatic Hospital, *Annual Report*, XXX (1862), 38–47; ibid., XXXI (1863), 32–33. Ray's brief remarks did not fully present his views. For a more sophisticated discussion see his paper "Management

of Hospitals for the Insane,'' originally written in 1863 as part of his annual report as superintendent of the Butler Hospital for the Insane and reprinted in *Contributions to Mental Pathology* (Boston, 1873, 391–408.

55. For a discussion of this debate see Grob, *Mental Institutions in America,* 304–19.

56. EJ, "Influence of Distance From and Nearness to an Insane Hospital on Its Use by the People,'' *American Journal of Insanity,* XXII (January 1866), 361–406; EJ to John P. Gray, February 26, March 13, 27, 1866, EJLB, CLMHMS; EJ, "Autobiography," 176, HLHU.

57. See Charles A. Lee to EJ, March 21, June 18, 27, 1866, March 12, 1867, EJ Papers, CLMHMS. Jarvis's obvious admiration of John Conolly can be gleaned from his appreciative article, "A Memoir of John Conolly, M.D., D.C.L.,'' *American Journal of Insanity,* XXVI (April 1870), 470–85.

58. John A. Andrew to EJ, June 1, 1864, EJ Papers, CFPL; EJ, "Connection of Intemperance with Disease and Mortality,'' *Boston Medical and Surgical Journal,* LXXIV (March 22, 1866), 149–54.

59. *Reports on the Subject of a License Law, by a Joint Special Committee of the Legislature of Massachusetts; Together with a Stenographic Report of the Testimony Taken Before Said Committee,* in Mass. *House Document No. 415* (May 14, 1867), passim; Boston *Daily Advertiser,* April 4, 1867; Henry G. Pearson, *The Life of John A. Andrew: Governor of Massachusetts 1861–1865* (2 vols.: Boston, 1904), II, 306ff.

60. *Reports on the Subject of a License Law,* 866–68.

61. Boston *Daily Advertiser,* April 4, 1867.

62. EJ to John A. Andrew, May 7, 1867, EJ to A.A. Miner, April 22, 1867, EJLB, CLMHMS. In the state elections in the fall of 1867 the supporters of licensing won a large majority. The licensing statute passed the following year (without the approval of the governor), however, was imperfectly drawn, leading to a reaction that resulted in a modified prohibition system. See *Acts and Resolves Passed by the General Court of Massachusetts, in the Year 1868* (Boston, 1868), 107–15, 325–26, and Pearson, *Life of John A. Andrew,* II, 309 n. 1.

63. *American Journal of Insanity,* XIX (July 1862), 71–72, 78–81.

64. EJ, "The Increase of Human Life,'' *Atlantic Monthly,* XXIV (October 1869), 495–506; ibid. (November 1869), 581–91; ibid. (December 1869), 711–18. This article was also circulated in pamphlet form. See EJ to Benjamin F. Stevens, July 19, 1871, EJ to F.S. Winston, January 23, 1872, EJLB, CLMHMS.

CHAPTER 8

1. "Records of the American Statistical Association 1839–1872," mss. vol., 67–68, ASA; EJ to Joseph C.G. Kennedy, August 26, 1859, EJLB, CLMHMS. As an example of the misuse of the statistics on insanity in the census of 1840 Jarvis cited Jean M.F.J. Boudin's *Traité de Géographie et de Statistique Médicales et des Maladies Endémiques* (2 vols.: Paris, 1857), which used the data from the sixth census.

2. EJ to Kennedy, October 20, 1859, February 21, 1860, EJLB, CLMHMS; Kennedy to EJ, March 19, 1860, EJ Papers, CLMHMS.

3. EJ to Kennedy, January 28, 1861, EJ to James Wynne, October 25, 1860, EJLB, CLMHMS.

4. EJ to Wynne, October 31, November 16, 1860, EJ to Kennedy, January 28, 1861, ibid.; Wynne to EJ, November 28, 1861, EJ Papers, CLMHMS; "Josiah Curtis 1816–1883," *Cosmos Club Bulletin,* XVII (May 1964), 3–4. In September 1861 Curtis, a long time acquaintance, informed Jarvis that Kennedy had received some communications from Wynne, but had neither recollections nor documentary evidence of Jarvis's plan. The only mention of the subject was Jarvis's letter to Kennedy of January 28, 1861, in which allusion was made to a more comprehensive proposal. Josiah Curtis to EJ, September 17, 1861, EJ Papers, CLMHMS.

5. Joseph C.G. Kennedy, *Preliminary Report on the Eighth Census. 1860* (Washington, D.C., 1862), 2–9, 22–32, 114–17, 138–67 (this report is also included in 37th Cong., 2d session, *House Executive Document No. 116* [1862]).

6. EJ to John Wingate Thornton, March 5, 1867, Department of Rare Books and Manuscripts, Boston Public Library, Boston, Mass.

7. EJ to John Wingate Thornton, February 28, 1867, ibid.; EJ to Henry G. Clarke, February 12, 1863, EJ to Kennedy, August 10, 1864, EJLB, CLMHMS.

8. Kennedy, *Preliminary Report on the Eighth Census,* 161; Wilson Jewell to EJ, August 25, October 5, 1863, EJ Papers, CLMHMS; EJ to Kennedy, June 1, August 4, September 7, 1863, February 4, 1864, March 7, 1865, EJLB, CLMHMS.

9. EJ to Kennedy, August 15, 1863, April 13, November 29, 1864, March 23, 1865, ibid.; EJ to John Wingate Thornton, February 28, 1867, Boston Public Library.

10. EJ to Kennedy, August 15, October 22, 1863, January 16, April 13, November 29, 1864, EJLB, CLMHMS. In a letter to Chadwick Jarvis specifically rejected a genetic explanation of the condition of the Irish and expressed the hope "that in another generation . . . this

new race will enjoy better health & more moral & intellectual vigor'' (EJ to Edwin Chadwick, June 10, 1853, ibid).

11. EJ to Kennedy, April 13, August 10, November 29, 1864, EJLB, CLMHMS.

12. EJ to Lord Carlisle, September 7, 1863, EJ to Salmon P. Chase, September 9, 1863, EJ to Kennedy, October 22, 1863, EJ to L.W. Meech, March 13, 1865, EJ to Frederic E. Winston, June 27, 1865, EJ to C.C. Coxe, October 15, 1865, ibid.; James Stark to EJ, June 20, 1865, EJ Papers, CLMHMS.

13. EJ to John Wingate Thornton, February 28, 1867, Boston Public Library; EJ to Kennedy, March 23, 1865, EJLB, CLMHMS.

14. EJ to Kennedy, March 7, 1865, EJLB, CLMHMS.

15. EJ to John Wingate Thornton, February 28, March 5, 1867, Boston Public Library; EJ to Kennedy, May 3, 1865, EJLB, CLMHMS; "Report of the Secretary of the Interior," in *Message of the President of the United States,* 39th Cong., 1st session, *House Executive Document No. 1* (December 4, 1865), xi; EJ, "Autobiography," 224–26, mss. vol., HLHU.

16. EJ to John Wingate Thornton, February 28, March 5, 1867, Boston Public Library; EJ to James Harlan, May or June ?, September 4, November 12, 1865, EJ to Henry Wilson, June 22, 1866, EJ to James S. Wilson, July 31, September 4, 23, October 12, 1865, April 23, May 18, 1867, EJ to Martha A. Cummins, November 11, 1865, EJ to J.M. Edmunds, July 8, September 4, October 2, 12, 29, 1865, EJLB, CLMHMS; EJ, "Autobiography," 229, HLHU.

17. Edwin M. Snow to EJ, August 12, 1865, EJ Papers, CLMHMS; James H. Cassedy, "Edwin Miller Snow: An Important American Public Health Pioneer," *Bulletin of the History of Medicine,* XXXV (March–April 1961), 156–62.

18. EJ to J.M. Edmunds, October 2, 12, 29, November 1, December 4, 1865, January 4, n.d. (beginning of April), May 2, 1866, EJ to James S. Wilson, November 1, n.d. (written between November 14 and 17), December 15, 1865, January 3, February 5, 19, 27, March 3, 26, 30, April 5, 14, 21, 27, 28, May 2, 19, 1866, EJ to James Harlan, November 18, 23, 1865, EJ to Charles Sumner, November 23, 1865, EJLB, CLMHMS.

19. *Statistics of the United States, (including Mortality, Property, &c.,) in 1860, Compiled from the Original Returns and Being the Final Exhibit of the Eighth Census* (Washington, D.C., 1866), xxiii–xxv.

20. Ibid., xxv–xxvi.

21. Ibid., xxvi–xliv. In newly settled states, where families tended

to be younger, there was a higher proportion of infants and children in the total population. This fact, insisted Jarvis, explained a good deal of the differences between Wisconsin and Texas on the one hand and Vermont and South Carolina on the other.

22. Ibid., xliv–xlix.

23. Ibid., l–lxvi.

24. EJ to Charles W. Elliott, January 20, 1868, EJLB, CLMHMS. See also EJ to J.W. [*sic., H.C.*] Lombard, August 10, 1867, ibid.

25. *Statistics of the United States . . . Being the Final Exhibit of the Eighth Census,* lxvii, 1–287.

26. Consider Jarvis's statistical work on the influence of occupation on longevity. Like most others of his age, he simply took crude occupational categories and age of death; from these he derived average longevity by occupation (see his paper "Connection of Occupation with Longevity," probably given before the members of the American Statistical Association about 1857 [copy in EJ Papers, CFPL]). Jarvis did not inquire into the total number of persons exposed to risk in particular occupations or the social and economic origins of its members, let alone other factors that might have a bearing on mortality patterns. Nor did he take into account the shortcomings of mortality reports.

27. 41st Cong., 1st session, *Congressional Globe,* 550–56. See also Garfield's address before the American Social Science Association on October 27, 1869, entitled "The American Census," *Journal of Social Science,* II (1870), 31–55.

28. Henry Villard to James A. Garfield, February 4, 1869, Garfield Papers, LC. As early as 1866 Jarvis urged the necessity of planning for the ninth census. See EJ to O.H. Browning, December 21, 1866, EJLB, CLMHMS.

29. Garfield to EJ, February 8, 1869, EJ to Garfield, February 15, 1869, Garfield Papers, LC. Garfield asked Jarvis to comment on the following: 1) whether the census could be better taken by internal revenue officials or marshalls; 2) whether changes should be made in regard to compensating census takers; 3) the time required to take the census; 4) modifications in the tables; 5) other suggestions.

30. EJ to Garfield, February 7, 1869, EJLB, CLMHMS, and reprinted in *Ninth Census. Communications from Dr. Franklin B. Hough and Others, Relative to the Ninth Census of the United States,* 41st Cong., 1st session, *House Miscellaneous Document No. 33* (April 1, 1869), 27–40.

31. EJ to Garfield, February 19, 1869, EJLB, CLMHMS, and reprinted in *Ninth Census. Communications from Dr. Franklin B. Hough and Others,* 37–40.

32. EJ to Garfield, February 23, March 1, 1869, EJLB, CLMHMS; *Ninth Census. Communications from Dr. Franklin B. Hough and Others,* 41–42; Garfield to EJ, February 22, 1869, Garfield Papers, LC.

33. Hough to EJ, March 1, 13, 22, 27, 1869, EJ Papers, CLMHMS. Garfield's correspondence supported Hough's observations on the difficulties of producing an accurate census. Indeed, one of the most significant problems grew out of the fear among many citizens that the enumerator was actually an assessor or tax-collector—a fear that resulted in deliberate misrepresentations. See H.S. Alden to Garfield, June 10, 1869, and Seth M. Dunning to Garfield, June 12, 1869, Garfield Papers, LC.

34. Hough to EJ, March 31, 1869, EJ Papers, CLMHMS; 41st Cong., 1st session, *Congressional Globe,* 249, 345, 491, 532, 540, 550–56.

35. Hough to EJ, April 10, 18, June 24, 1869, Edwin B. Snow to EJ, April 15, 1869, EJ Papers, CLMHMS; Henry Villard to Garfield, April 22, May 5, 27, June 15, 1869, EJ to Garfield, May 26, June 3, 1869, Garfield to EJ, July 19, 1869, Garfield Papers, LC; EJ to William Farr, May 1, 1869, EJ to Garfield, May 11, 1869, EJ to Hough, June 21, 1869, EJ to Charles Sumner, June 23, 1869, EJLB, CLMHMS; *American Journal of Insanity,* XXVI (October 1869), 179–81.

36. Hough to EJ, June 24, July 12, 14, September 1, 1869, EJ Papers, CLMHMS.

37. Garfield to EJ, July 19, December 9, 1869, George N. Rose to Garfield, July 7, 12, 1869, Garfield Papers, LC; EJ to Garfield, December 29, 1869, EJLB, CLMHMS; "Ninth Census," 41st Cong., 2d session, *House Report No. 3* (January 18, 1870), Appendix C (by EJ), 99–120.

38. Garfield to Halsey R.W. Hall, January 25, 1870, Garfield Papers, LC; 41st Cong., 2d session, *Congressional Globe,* 183, 238, 267–68, et passim.

39. Edwin M. Snow to Garfield, December 9, 1869, January 18, 1870, Garfield to Snow, January 20, 1870, Garfield Papers, LC; EJ to Henry Wilson, January 22, 29, 1870, EJLB, CLMHMS; Snow to EJ, February 16, 1870, EJ Papers, CLMHMS; 41st Cong., 2d session, *Congressional Globe,* 267–68, 1039, 1078, 1103, 1131–48; James P. Munroe, *A Life of Francis Amasa Walker* (New York, 1923), 110ff.; "The United States Census of 1870," *Journal of Social Science,* III (1871), 223–26. Henry Adams attributed the defeat of the Garfield bill to a combination of personal antagonism between Conkling and Charles Sumner, and an intense rivalry between the House and Senate for power ("The Census Imbroglio," *The Nation,* X (February 24, 1870), 116–17).

40. 41st Cong., 2d session, *Congressional Globe,* 2121, 2125, 2561, 2708-9, 2942, 3174-75, 3203, 3242; Garfield to Walker, May 4, 1870, Garfield Papers, LC; EJ to Garfield, March 16, 1870, Garfield Papers, LC and EJLB, CLMHMS.

41. EJ to Walker, February or March, 1870, November 24, 1871, EJLB, CLMHMS; EJ, "Autobiography," 237, HLHU. Jarvis encountered some problems in collecting compensation for his work for the Garfield committee, but by the end of the summer of 1870 the difficulties were resolved. See EJ to Oakes Ames, June 19, 22, 1870, EJ to Garfield, June 22, 1870, EJ to William A. Richardson, August 1, 8, 1870, EJ to George S. Boutwell, August 1, 1870, EJLB, CLMHMS.

42. *The Statistics of the Population of the United States* (Ninth Census, vol. I) (Washington, D.C., 1872), xixff.; *The Vital Statistics of the United States* (Ninth Census, vol. II) (Washington, D.C., 1872), ix.

43. In 1873 Jarvis wrote the article on the census for *Appleton's Encyclopedia.* See Eton Sylvester Drone to EJ, May 3, 1873, James Reed Chadwick Papers, CLMHMS.

CHAPTER 9

1. EJ, "Autobiography," 47, mss., HLHU.

2. Ibid., 212-15; EJ to Rev. George Garrett, September 14, October 1, 1870, November 23, 1871, EJ to Charles E. Stedman, January 14, 1870, EJLB, CLMHMS; Elisha Harris to EJ, January 25, 1873, EJ Papers, CLMHMS; *Reports and Papers Presented at the Meetings of the American Public Health Association in the Years 1874-1875* (New York, 1876), 537; *Journal of Social Science,* VII (September 1874), 229-34.

3. Jarvis was appalled at the high death rate at state almshouses. In his testimony before the committee he conceded that many of the children came from degraded parents but questioned whether the state was doing enough to rescue them from death by providing food, care, and air. The legislative committee concurred with the petitioners and urged the legislature to establish a separate foundling hospital at the state almshouse in Bridgewater. Only the determined opposition of Franklin B. Sanborn, the influential secretary of the board of state charities, prevented favorable action. See *Medical Communications of the Massachusetts Medical Society,* 2d ser. VII (Boston, 1874), 52-53, 55-56; Mass. *House Document No. 44* (February 1868), 1-2; Mass.

Senate Document No. 294 (May 21, 1868), 1–19; Mass. Board of State Charities, *Annual Report*, V (1868), 74–75.

4. Mass. *Senate Document No. 340* (May 22, 1869), 1–6.

5. Barbara G. Rosenkrantz, *Public Health and the State: Changing Views in Massachusetts, 1842-1936* (Cambridge, 1972), chap. 2. For Bowditch's views see his *Public Hygiene in America* (Boston, 1877), and Vincent Y. Bowditch, *Life and Correspondence of Henry Ingersoll Bowditch by His Son* (2 vols.: Boston, 1902), II, 217ff.

6. Henry I. Bowditch to EJ, May 18, 1869, EJ Papers, CLMHMS.

7. Rosenkrantz, *Public Health and the State*, chap. 2.

8. Bowditch to EJ, October 5, 1869, EJ Papers, CLMHMS; EJ to Bowditch, December 17, 1869, EJLB, CLMHMS.

9. EJ, "Infant Mortality," Mass. State Board of Health, *Annual Report*, IV (1872), 192–233, and "Political Economy of Health," ibid., V (1873), 333–90; George Derby to EJ, April 20, December 23, 1872, January 19, 1873, Edwin Chadwick to EJ, August 24, 1874, EJ Papers, CLMHMS.

10. EJ, "Political Economy of Health," 371.

11. EJ, "Relation of Education to Insanity," in *Report of the Commissioner of Education for the Year 1871* (Washington, D.C., 1872), 538–46; EJ, "The Value of Common-School Education to Common Labor," in *Report of the Commissioner of Education for the Year 1872* (Washington, D.C., 1873), 572–85, and reissued in *Circulars of Information of the Bureau of Education*, no. 3 (1879), 215–52; EJ to John Eaton, December 25, 1871, EJLB, CLMHMS; Eaton to EJ, January 24, February 13, April 29, September 7, 1872, EJ Papers, CLMHMS.

12. American Social Science Association, *Document Published by the Association with an Abridgement of the Transactions* (Part I–II: Boston, 1866–1867), 1–34; *Journal of Social Science*, I (June 1869), 1. See also Harold M. Hyman, *A More Perfect Union: The Impact of the Civil War and Reconstruction on the Constitution* (New York, 1973), 311–12; John G. Sproat, *"The Best Men": Liberal Reformers in the Gilded Age* (New York, 1968), 56–57 et passim; L.L. Bernard and Jessie Bernard, *Origins of American Sociology: The Social Science Movement in the United States* (New York, 1943), 527ff; Mary O. Furner, *Advocacy & Objectivity: A Crisis in the Professionalization of American Social Science, 1865-1905* (Lexington, 1975), 10–34.

13. *Journal of Social Science*, I (June 1869), 195; ibid., II (1870), vi; EJ, "Autobiography," 241–42, HLHU; Sproat, *"The Best Men,"* 57; EJ to David W. Lincoln, November 9, 1870, EJLB, CLMHMS. The most authoritative history of the American Social Science Association

is Thomas L. Haskell's "Safe Haven for Sound Opinion: The American Social Science Association and the Professionalization of Social Thought in the United States, 1865–1909" (Ph.D. diss., Stanford University, 1972).

14. Kapp came to the United States from Germany after the abortive revolutions of 1848 and became a leading figure in New York City literary and political circles. His paper dealt with immigration to the United States; it demonstrated little overt hostility toward immigrants. Indeed, he opposed federal regulation and argued that rapid American economic growth was in large measure attributable to a high rate of immigration. See Kapp, "Immigration," *Journal of Social Science,* II (1870), 1–30.

15. Ibid., 16–18.

16. Francis A. Walker, "Our Population in 1900," *Atlantic Monthly,* XXXII (October 1873), 487–95; idem., "American Irish and American Germans," *Scribner's Monthly,* VI (June 1873), 172–79; idem., "Occupations and Mortality of Our Foreign Population, 1870," *Chicago Advance,* November 12, December 10, 1874, January 14, 1875, reprinted in *Discussions in Economics and Statistics,* ed. Davis R. Dewey (2 vols.: New York, 1899), II, 213–22; *The Statistics of the Population of the United States* (Ninth Census, vol. I) (Washington, D.C., 1872), xviii–xix; Barbara M. Solomon, *Ancestors and Immigrants: A Changing New England Tradition* (Cambridge, 1956), 69ff.

17. Jarvis wrote to David A. Wells to get additional data; he also contacted Garfield and expressed the hope that the new census would rectify such misconceptions (EJ to David A. Wells, November 25, 1869, EJLB, CLMHMS; EJ to James A. Garfield, December 4, 1869, Garfield Papers, LC [copy in EJLB, CLMHMS]).

18. A German immigrant who worked briefly in the census department in the mid-1850s, Schade published a pamphlet entitled *The Immigration into the United States of America, from a Statistical and National-Economical Point of View* (Washington, D.C., 1856). Schade's pamphlet bitterly castigated the Know-Nothing movement, portrayed the positive contributions of immigrants, and rejected estimates that immigrants would overshadow natives.

19. EJ to Francis A. Walker, February 3, April 15, 1871, EJ to E.B. Elliott, April 15, 1871, EJLB, CLMHMS; EJ, "Immigration," *Atlantic Monthly,* XXIX (April 1872), 454–68.

20. EJ, "Immigration," *Atlantic Monthly,* XXIX (April 1872), 466–68. In another paper prepared for the eighth International Statistical Congress in Russia in 1872 (which he did not attend), Jarvis sum-

marized all of his findings about the history of the progress of the American population. His tone again remained neutral; he drew no invidious conclusions. Only in his discussion of the Indian population did a note of pessimism appear; he feared that the unwillingness of the Indians to adopt the more civilized ways of white society would hasten their disappearance. See EJ, "History of the Progress of Population of the United States of North America," in *Congrès International de Statistique, Compte-Rendu de la Huitième Session a St-Pétersbourg* (3 vols.: St-Pétersbourg, 1874), III, 1–9. This was also reprinted in the transactions of the American Statistical Association and circulated in pamphlet form (Boston, 1877). Jarvis unsuccessfully attempted to become the official American delegate to the seventh Congress held at the Hague in 1869; he also expressed the desire to attend the eighth in 1872. See EJ to Charles Sumner, April 5, 10, 1869, Sumner Papers, HLHU (copies in EJLB, CLMHMS); Sumner to EJ, April 7, 14, 1869, EJ Papers, CLMHMS; EJ to George S. Boutwell, April 5, 1869, EJ to Dr. von Bauenhauer, April ?, 1870, EJ to Pierre Simenow, February 2, 1875, EJLB, CLMHMS.

21. EJ, "Vital Statistics of Different Races," *Journal of Social Science,* VII (September 1874), 229–34.

22. Jarvis to Walker, May 11, 1875, EJLB, CLMHMS.

23. EJ to Joseph Henry, December 4, 1872, Henry Papers, Smithsonian Institution, Washington, D.C.

24. Barbara G. Rosenkrantz, "Cart Before Horse: Theory, Practice and Professional Image in American Public Health, 1870–1920," *Journal of the History of Medicine and Allied Sciences,* XXIX (January 1974), 55–73.

25. Elisha Harris to EJ, January 25, 1873, EJ Papers, CLMHMS; *Reports and Papers Presented at the Meetings of the American Public Health Association in the Years 1874-1875,* 533, 536–37, 539–40; EJ, "Autobiography," 210–13, HLHU (his discussion of women in his autobiography was probably identical with the paper presented before the association). Lucy Sewall on several occasions called upon Jarvis for help; in 1873 she asked him to aid a female physician being considered for membership in the Massachusetts Medical Society. See Sewall to EJ, May 12, 1867, February 4, 1873, EJ Papers, CLMHMS.

26. This description is taken from *Report of the Trial of Samuel M. Andrews, Indicted for the Murder of Cornelius Holmes, Before the Supreme Judicial Court of Massachusetts, December 11, 1868* (New York, 1869), and EJ, "Trial of Samuel M. Andrews for the Murder of Cornelius Holmes," *American Journal of Insanity,* XXVI (April 1870), 385–407.

27. *Report of the Trial of Samuel M. Andrews,* 99–122, 172–84, 186–90, 223–35, 252–60; EJ to Charles G. Davis, February 4, December 24, 1869, December 2, 1870, EJLB, CLMHMS. As an expert witness, Jarvis received $50 per diem from the court (the established rate recommended by the Massachusetts Medical Society).

28. *Report of the Trial of Samuel M. Andrews,* 222–35, 252–60.

29. EJ to Pliny Earle, sheet attached to a letter dated October 13, 1864, but obviously written in 1869, Earle Papers, AAS; EJ to Luther Parker, Jr., February 1, 1869, EJLB, CLMHMS; EJ, "Mania Transitoria," *Boston Medical and Surgical Journal,* n.s. III (June 10, 1869), 329–37 (June 17, 1869), 353–57, and the *American Journal of Insanity,* XXVI (July 1869), 1–32 (also reprinted in *Report of the Trial of Samuel M. Andrews,* 265–86); EJ, "Trial of Samuel M. Andrews for Murder," *Boston Medical and Surgical Journal,* n.s. IV (November 4, 1869), 237–45, and (with a slightly different title) in the *American Journal of Insanity,* XXVI (April 1870), 385–407.

30. *Report of the Trial of Samuel M. Andrews,* 172–85, 222–35, 286–87. See also Charles E. Rosenberg, *The Trial of the Assassin Guiteau: Psychiatry and Law in the Gilded Age* (Chicago, 1968), and David Brion Davis, *Homicide in American Fiction, 1798–1860: A Study in Social Values* (Ithaca, 1957), chaps. 3–4.

31. *American Journal of Insanity,* XXIX (October 1872), 140–66; EJ to James D. Calt, August 25, 1870, EJLB, CLMHMS.

32. On this conflict see Gerald N. Grob, *Mental Institutions in America: Social Policy to 1875* (New York, 1973), chap. 7, and *The State and the Mentally Ill: A History of Worcester State Hospital in Massachusetts, 1830–1920* (Chapel Hill, 1966), chap. 6.

33. John Curwen to EJ, July 19, 1870, EJ Papers, CLMHMS; EJ to Henry I. Bowditch, September 26, 1871, EJLB, CLMHMS; *American Journal of Insanity,* XXVIII (October 1871), 337; EJ, "Proper Provision for the Insane," in Mass. State Board of Health, *Annual Report,* III (1871), 139–59.

34. EJ, "Proper Provision for the Insane," 139–59.

35. See Grob, *Mental Institutions in America,* 263ff.

36. *American Journal of Insanity,* XXVIII (October 1871), 320–40.

37. Northampton State Lunatic Hospital, *Annual Report,* XVII (1872), 36–42; Ray to Earle, February 18, 1872, Kirkbride to Earle, March 3, 1873, Earle Papers, AAS; Ray to John Sawyer, February 15, 1873, Butler Hospital Library, Providence, Rhode Island; EJ to Merrick Bemis, January 29, 1870, EJLB, CLMHMS. For this controversy see Grob, *Mental Institutions in America,* chaps. 7–8.

38. Julius Parigot to EJ, n.d., EJ Papers, CLMHMS. See Parigot's

earlier article, "The Gheel Question: From an American Point of View," *American Journal of Insanity,* XIX (January 1863), 332–54.

39. For the favorable reception of Jarvis's plan for uniform statistics at this meeting see the *American Journal of Insanity,* XXVIII (October 1871), 213, 280–319.

40. EJ, "Autobiography," HLHU.

41. See the critical comments of Willard Parker, who questioned the emphasis in medical schools on treatment and cure (as compared with prevention), in Willard Parker to EJ, December 18, 1871, EJ Papers, CLMHMS.

42. Edwin M. Snow to EJ, July 24, 1874, Kirkbride to EJ, March 2, 1875, ibid. See also Elisha Harris to EJ, August 31, 1874, Snow to EJ, November 19, 1874, ibid.; Almira Jarvis to George Ripley, March 6, 1874, Almira Jarvis to Amory Starr, May 22, June 11, 1874, EJ to Henry Adams, May 10, 1875, EJ to A.J. Johnson, September, 1876, October 5, 1876, EJ to A.S. Barnes, November 23, 1876, EJLB, CLMHMS.

43. See EJ's annotated copy of Lemuel Shattuck's *A History of the Town of Concord* (Boston, 1835), CFPL; EJ, "Traditions and Reminiscences of Concord Massachusetts, or a Contribution to the Social and Domestic History of the Town 1779 to 1878," v–viii, mss., CFPL; EJ, "Deaths Concord Mass. 1779 to 1878," mss., CFPL; EJ to George A. Jarvis, January 21, July 22, 1878, EJLB, CLMHMS.

44. EJ, "Traditions and Reminiscences," 184–99, 390–465, et passim, CFPL. The sections dealing with liquor were read in abridged form before the American Statistical Association in 1882 and published in pamphlet form, *Financial Condition of the Use of Spirits and Wine With the People of Concord, Massachusetts* (Boston, 1883). Jarvis's concern with intemperance was reflected in his European correspondence. See Achille Foville to EJ, August 13, 1871, February 27, June 27, 1872, March 12, 1873 (translation), EJLB, CLMHMS; J.G. Varrentrepp to EJ, August 9, 1872, March 9, 1873, Abraham A. Baer to EJ, January 14, 1873, EJ Papers, CLMHMS.

45. EJ, "Houses & People. Concord Mass. 1810–1820," mss., CFPL.

46. Ibid.; EJ, "The Supposed Decay of Families," *New England Historical and Genealogical Register,* XXXVIII (October 1884), 385–95, also circulated in pamphlet form under the title *Supposed Decay of Families in New England Disproved by the Experience of the People of Concord, Mass.* (Boston, 1884).

47. John Curwen to EJ, May 11, 1876, EJ Papers, CLMHMS; EJ to George [?], May 12, 1877, EJ to John Trowbridge, May 15, 1879, EJLB,

CLMHMS; "Record Book. American Statistical Association. 1872–1916," 75–76, mss., ASA.

48. Willard Parker to EJ, October 26, 1879, March 13, 1880, EJ Papers, CLMHMS; EJ to the Committee of the Directory for Nurses, March 25, 1881, EJLB, CLMHMS; Boston *Evening Transcript*, November 3, 1884; Edward Jarvis Will (No. 72,319) and Almira Jarvis Will (No. 72,320), Suffolk County Probate Court, Boston, Mass.; John S. Keyes, "Memoir of Edward Jarvis," in *Memoirs of Members of the Social Circle in Concord: Second Series from 1795 to 1840* (Cambridge, 1888), 352–53.

49. "Undivided Lives," *Christian Register*, LXIII (November 6, 1884), 706.

50. EJ, "Cookery and Health," *Unitarian Review and Religious Magazine*, XXII (November 1884), 401–16.

51. Andrew P. Peabody, "Memoir of Edward Jarvis, M.D.," *New England Historical and Genealogical Register*, XXXIX (July 1885), 217–24; Robert W. Wood, *Memorial of Edward Jarvis, M.D.* (Boston, 1885); "Edward Jarvis, M.D.," American Antiquarian Society, *Proceedings*, n.s. III (October 1883—April 1885), 484–87; "Edward Jarvis," American Academy of Arts and Sciences, *Proceedings*, n.s. XII (1884–1885), 519–22; *Boston Medical and Surgical Journal*, CXI (December 18, 1884), 598–99; Keyes, "Memoir of Edward Jarvis," 317–55.

W.A.F. Browne, the distinguished British psychiatrist, noted in 1881 that Jarvis "who, though not as great a man as [Isaac] Ray was even a greater worker." In making this observation Browne captured an important element of truth about Jarvis's career. See Browne to Thomas S. Kirkbride, November 11, 1881, Kirkbride Papers, IPH. See also G. Alder Blumer, "A Half-Century of American Medico-Psychological Literature," American Medico-Psychological Association, *Proceedings*, I (1894), 151–52.

52. Peabody, "Memoir of Edward Jarvis, M.D.," 219–20. See also Barbara G. Rosenkrantz's paper, "The Search for Professional Order in 19th Century American Medicine," which was delivered at the Fourteenth International Congress of the History of Science, Tokyo, Japan, 1974.

Selected
Bibliography

MANUSCRIPTS

Boston, Massachusetts

—*Boston Public Library*
Department of Rare Books and Manuscripts, miscellaneous items,
catalogued separately.
—*Countway Library of Medicine, Harvard Medical School*
James Read Chadwick Papers.
William Cranch Bond Fifield Papers.
James Jackson Papers.
Edward Jarvis, "Concord to Louisville 1837" (a journal).
Edward Jarvis Letter Books (10 vols., May 1843 – July 1884; volume
II, covering August 1850 – February 1853, is missing).
Edward Jarvis Papers.
Benjamin Lincoln Papers.
Miscellaneous Manuscripts, from Boston Medical Library.
"Report of the Physicians of Massachusetts. Superintendents of
Hospitals. . . . and Others Describing the Insane and Idiotic Per-
sons in the State of Massachusetts in 1855. Made to the Commis-
sioners on Lunacy."
—*Massachusetts Archives, State House*
Miscellaneous items.
—*Massachusetts Historical Society*
John A. Andrew Papers.
Henry W. Bellows Papers.
Charles Deane Papers.
Samuel A. Green Papers.

Horace Mann Papers.
Lemuel Shattuck Papers.
John C. Warren Papers.
Joseph E. Worcester Papers.
—*Suffolk County Probate Court*
Edward Jarvis Will (No. 72,319) and Almira Jarvis Will (No. 72,320).

Brussels, Belgium

—*Academie royale de Belgique*
Correspondence of A. Quetelet

Cambridge, Massachusetts

—*Middlesex County Probate Court*
Probate record of estate of Francis Jarvis (died intestate in 1840).
—*Harvard University Archives*
Edward Jarvis, "Harvard College. Account of Class of 1826."
Harvard College Papers, 2d series, XXX (1863), 81–82.
Manuscript notes of Library Committee meeting, December 26,
1863, Jarvis Quinquennial folder.
—*Harvard University, Houghton Library*
John P. Bigelow Papers.
Francis William Bird Papers.
Dorothea L. Dix Papers.
Ralph Waldo Emerson Papers.
Samuel Gridley Howe Papers.
Edward Jarvis, "Autobiography."
George Nichols Papers.
John Gorham Palfrey Papers.
Charles Sumner Papers.

Concord, Massachusetts

—*Concord Free Public Library*
Concord Lyceum Manuscript Records (6 vols.).
Concord Town Records (microfilm).
Edward Jarvis, Diary (vol. I listed as "Autobiography"; vol. II as the
"Private Journal of Edward Jarvis").
Edward Jarvis, "Deaths Concord Mass. 1779 to 1878."
Edward Jarvis, "European Letters" (3 vols.).
Edward Jarvis, "Houses & People. Concord. Mass. 1810–1820."
Edward Jarvis, "Traditions and Reminiscences of Concord Massa-
chusetts, or a Contribution to the Social and Domestic History of
the Town 1779 to 1878."

Ezra Ripley, "An Account of Deaths in the Town of Concord from the Year 1778 [to 1857]."

Ezra Ripley, "Ezra Ripley's Book Containing an Account of Marriages Solemnized by him from November 11, 1778 to December 21, 1840."

Lemuel Shattuck, *A History of the Town of Concord.* Boston and Concord: Russell, Odiorne and Co., 1835. This edition contains Edward Jarvis's manuscript notes and addendum.

Durham, North Carolina

—*Perkins Library, Duke University*
James D.B. De Bow Papers.

New York, New York

—*New York Public Library*
United States Sanitary Commission Papers.

Philadelphia, Pennsylvania

—*Institute of the Pennsylvania Hospital*
Thomas S. Kirkbride Papers.

Providence, Rhode Island

—*Isaac Ray Medical Library, Butler Hospital*
Miscellaneous letter collection.

San Marino, California

—*Henry E. Huntington Library*
Ward Hill Lamon Papers.
Francis Lieber Papers.
William Jones Rhees Papers.
Caleb B. Smith – Charles W. Spooner Papers.

Washington, D.C.

—*American Statistical Association*
"Clippings of the American Statistical Association."
"Record Book. American Statistical Association. 1872–1916."
"Records of the American Statistical Association 1839–1872."
"Records of the Board of Directors of the American Statistical Association in Boston."

—*Library of Congress*
James A. Garfield Papers.
Walter Willcox Papers.

—*National Archives*
  Records of the Bureau of the Census, Record Group 20.
—*Smithsonian Institution*
  Joseph Henry Papers.

Waverly, Massachusetts

—*Walter E. Fernald State School*
  Manuscript records of the Massachusetts School for Idiotic and
  Feebleminded Youth.

Worcester, Massachusetts

—*American Antiquarian Society*
  George Chandler Papers.
  Pliny Earle Papers.
  Samuel B. Woodward Papers.

PUBLISHED WORKS OF EDWARD JARVIS
(Listed chronologically)

"Account of a Remarkable Epidemic in Warwick, Mass." *Medical
  Magazine,* I (February 1833), 449–54.
"Ladies' Fairs." *New England Magazine,* V (July 1833), 54–59.
"Intemperance and Disease." *Boston Medical and Surgical Journal,*
  XV (November 30, 1836), 261–67.
Letters from Louisville. Published in the *Yeoman's Gazette* (Concord),
  July 31, 1837, February 24, March 31, November 24, December 1,
  1838; *The Republican,* July 30, 1841.
"True Delicacy Toward Animals." *Western Messenger,* VI (November
  1838), 19–24.
"Kentucky Historical Society." *Western Messenger,* VI (November
  1838), 61–62.
"Mr. Young's Discourse on the Life and Character of Dr. Bowditch."
  Western Messenger, VI (November 1838), 63–66.
"Sunday Schools in Louisville." *Western Messenger,* VI (November
  1838), 144.
"New-England Non-Resistance Society." *Western Messenger,* VIII
  (September 1840), 193–201.
"Insanity in Kentucky." *Boston Medical and Surgical Journal,* XXIV
  (April 21, 1841), 165–71.
Insanity and Insane Asylums. Louisville: Prentice and Weissinger,

1841. Also published as a review article in the *Western Journal of Medicine and Surgery,* IV (December 1841), 443–82.

What Shall We Do with the Insane of the Western Country? Louisville: n.p., 1842. Also published as "What Shall We Do with Our Insane?" *Western Journal of Medicine and Surgery,* V (February 1842), 81–125.

"Prospects of the Blind and Insane in Kentucky." *Boston Medical and Surgical Journal,* XXVI (March 2, 1842), 60–61.

"Insane Asylums in the West." *Boston Medical and Surgical Journal,* XXVI (March 23, 1842), 101–6.

"Some Account of the Kentucky Historical Society." *American Quarterly Register,* XV (August 1842), 72–77.

"Statistics of Insanity in the United States." *Boston Medical and Surgical Journal,* XXVII (September 21, 1842), 116–21, and (November 30, 1842), 281–82.

"Sixth Annual Report of the Board of Education. With the Sixth Annual Report of the Secretary of the Board." *Christian Examiner,* XXXIV (July 1843), 366–81.

"Law of Physical Life." *Christian Examiner,* XXXV (September, 1843), 1–31.

"Insanity Among the Coloured Population of the Free States." *American Journal of the Medical Sciences,* n.s. VII (January 1844), 71–83.

[Edward Jarvis, William Brigham, and J. Wingate Thornton]. "Memorial of the American Statistical Association, Praying the Adoption of Measures for the Correction of Errors in the Returns of the Sixth Census." 28th Cong., 2d session, *Senate Document No. 5* (December 10, 1844).

"Chadwick on the Practice of Interment in Towns." *American Journal of the Medical Sciences,* IX (January 1845), 131–54.

[Edward Jarvis, J. Wingate Thornton, and William Brigham]. "The Sixth Census of the United States." *Hunt's Merchants' Magazine,* XII (February 1845), 125–39.

"Dunglison on Human Health." *American Journal of the Medical Sciences,* n.s. IX (April 1845), 379–90.

Lecture on the Necessity of the Study of Physiology, Delivered Before the American Institute of Instruction. at Hartford, August 22, 1845. Boston: William D. Ticknor & Co., 1845.

"Notice of Some Vital Statistics of the United States, in a Letter to the Hon. Horace Mann, by MR. EDWARD JARVIS, of Dorchester, Massachusetts, United States, dated 22nd April, 1845. Abstracted and Compared with the Statistics of England and Wales. By THOS. LAYCOCK, M.D." *Journal of the Statistical Society of London,* IX (October 1846), 277–79.

[Edward Jarvis et al.]. "Petition of the American Statistical Association [for a Sanitary Survey of the State]." Mass. *House Document No. 16* (February 9, 1848).

Practical Physiology; For the Use of Schools and Families. Philadelphia: Thomas, Cowperthwait, & Co., 1847, 1848. A very slightly revised edition, which included seventy engravings, was published in 1852 under the title *Practical Physiology; Or, Anatomy and Physiology Applied to Health. For the Use of Schools and Families.* Philadelphia: Thomas, Cowperthwait & Co., 1852. The last edition appeared in 1866 under the title *Physiology and Laws of Health. For the Use of Schools, Academies, and Colleges.* New York: A.S. Barnes & Co., 1866.

Primary Physiology, for Schools. Philadelphia: Thomas, Cowperthwait & Co., 1848, 1850.

"Sanitary Reform." *American Journal of the Medical Sciences,* XV (April 1848), 419–50.

"County Receptacles for the Insane." Boston *Daily Journal,* March 12, 1849.

"Reports on Idiocy." *American Journal of the Medical Sciences,* n.s. XVII (April 1849), 421–41. Also reprinted as "Causes, Cure, and Prevention of Idiocy." *Journal of Psychological Medicine and Mental Pathology,* III (July 1, 1850), 292–322.

"Treatises on Ventilation." *American Journal of the Medical Sciences,* n.s. XVIII (July 1849), 129–47.

[Edward Jarvis, John D. Fisher, and S. Parkman]. Letter to Lemuel Shattuck, December 10, 1849. In *Report of a General Plan for the Promotion of Public and Personal Health, Devised, Prepared and Recommended by the Commissioners Appointed Under a Resolve of the Legislature of Massachusetts, Relating to a Sanitary Survey of the State. Presented April 25, 1850.* Boston: Dutton & Wentworth, 1850, 352–58.

"Sanitary Condition of Massachusetts and New England." American Medical Association. *Transactions,* III (1850), 247–66.

"The Influence of Distance From and Proximity to an Insane Hospital, on its Use by Any People." *Boston Medical and Surgical Journal,* XLII (April 17, 1850), 209–22. Partly reprinted in *American Journal of Insanity,* VII (January 1851), 281–85.

"On the Comparative Liability of Males and Females to Insanity, and

Their Comparative Curability and Mortality When Insane." *American Journal of Insanity,* VII (October 1850), 142–71.

"Report of the Sanitary Commission of Massachusetts." *Boston Medical and Surgical Journal,* XLIV (March 5, 1851), 89–97.

[Review of the *Report of the Sanitary Commission of Massachusetts*]. *American Journal of the Medical Sciences,* XXI (April 1851), 391–409.

"Plan and Structure of Insane Hospitals." *Boston Medical and Surgical Journal,* XLIV (July 23, 1851), 494–95.

"Causes of Insanity." *Boston Medical and Surgical Journal,* XLV (November 12, 1851), 289–305. Also circulated in pamphlet form as *On the Causes of Insanity.* N.p.: n.p., n.d. (c. 1851).

"Insanity Among the Coloured Population of the Free States." *American Journal of Insanity,* VIII (January 1852), 268–82.

"The Massachusetts General Hospital." *Christian Examiner,* LII (March 1852), 215–25.

"On the Supposed Increase of Insanity." *American Journal of Insanity,* VIII (April 1852), 333–64.

"The Late Dr. Robert Thaxter, of Dorchester." *Boston Medical and Surgical Journal,* XLVI (May 19, 1852), 309–14.

"Births, Marriages, and Deaths in Massachusetts." *American Journal of the Medical Sciences,* XXIV (July 1852), 147–64.

Memoir of the Life and Character of George Cheyne Shattuck, M.D. N.p.: n.p., n.d. (c. 1854).

"Memoir of Francis Jarvis." In *Memoirs of Members of the Social Circle in Concord: Second Series from 1795 to 1840.* Cambridge: Riverside Press, 1888, 30–51. (Written in 1854.)

"The Production of Vital Force." In *Medical Communications of the Massachusetts Medical Society,* 2d ser. vol. IV. Boston: Massachusetts Medical Society, 1854. Pp. 1–40.

"Registration of Births, Marriages, and Deaths." *American Journal of the Medical Sciences,* XXIX (April 1855), 407–30.

Report on Insanity and Idiocy in Massachusetts, by the Commission on Lunacy, Under Resolve of the Legislature of 1854. Mass. *House Document No. 144* (1855).

Mass. *House Document No. 282* (April 26, 1855). This committee report was written by Jarvis.

Rules and Regulations of the Board of Health of the Town of Dorchester, Massachusetts. Adopted, August 15th, 1855. Dorchester: Gazette and Chronicle Press, 1855.

"Letter from Dr. Edward Jarvis, of Massachusetts, Upon the Classification of Diseases" (September 22, 1855). In *Mortality Statistics of the Seventh Census of the United States, 1850,* 33rd Cong., 2d sess., *House Executive Document No. 98.* Washington, D.C.: A.O.P. Nicholson, 1855. Pp. 45–48.

"To the Medical Profession of Massachusetts." *Boston Medical and Surgical Journal,* LIII (November 22, 1855), 337–42.

Address Delivered at the Laying of the Corner Stone of the Insane Hospital, at Northampton, Massachusetts. Northampton: J. & L. Metcalf, 1856.

"The Influence of Occupations Upon Health." *Boston Medical and Surgical Journal,* LIV (July 24, 1856), 505–7.

"Connection of Occupation with Longevity." One-page printed sheet, c. 1857. Copy in Jarvis Papers, CFPL.

"Obituary of Samuel Hoar." *Christian Examiner,* LXII (January 1857), 154–60.

"Criminal Insane. Insane Transgressors and Insane Convicts." *American Journal of Insanity,* XIII (January 1857), 195–231.

"Distribution of Lunatic Hospital Reports." *American Journal of Insanity,* XIV (January 1858), 248–53.

"Report on Registration of Births, Marriages, and Deaths." American Medical Association. *Transactions,* XI (1858), 525–47.

"Tendency of Misdirected Education and the Unbalanced Mind to Produce Insanity." *American Journal of Education,* IV (March 1858), 591–612. Also reprinted in *Journal of Psychological Medicine and Mental Pathology,* XI (July 1, 1858), 424–44.

Two letters to George H. Snelling, March 30, 1857, April 2, 1859. In Mass. *Senate Document No. 186* (April 1859), 10–16.

Review of James Wynne, *Report on the Vital Statistics of the United States, Made to the Mutual Life Insurance Company of New York* (New York: H. Bailliere, 1857). In *American Journal of the Medical Sciences,* XXVII (April 1859), 458–86.

"Causes of Mental Disease." *North American Review,* LXXXIX (October 1859), 316–39.

"Law of Insanity, and Hospitals for the Insane in Massachusetts." *Monthly Law Reporter,* XXII (November 1859), 385–409.

"On the Proper Functions of Private Institutions or Homes for the Insane." *American Journal of Insanity,* XVII (July 1860), 19–31. Also reprinted in part in *Journal of Psychological Medicine and Mental Pathology,* XIII (October 1, 1860), 596–600.

"On the System of Taxation Prevailing in the United States, and Especially in Massachusetts." *Journal of the Statistical Society of London,* XXIII (September 1860), 370–78.

"Vital Statistics of the United States of America"; "Connection of Occupation with Longevity"; "Comparative Liability of Males and Females to Various Kinds of Crime"; and "Some Suggestions for Further Inquiry as to Vital Statistics in the Census Enumeration." All in *Report of the Proceedings of the Fourth Session of the International Statistical Congress, Held in London July 16th, and the Five Following Days.* London: Her Majesty's Stationary Office, 1861. Pp. 51–55, 271–72, 446–47, 497–99.

[Edward Jarvis, Josiah Quincy, Jr., and Josiah Curtis]. "Memorial of the Boston Sanitary Association to the Legislature of Massachusetts, Asking for the Establishment of a Board of Health and of Vital Statistics." Mass. *House Document No. 112* (February 15, 1861).

"Petition of Edw'd Jarvis, Sam'l G. Howe, and C.C. Felton, Praying the Establishment of a Board of Health for the Army." 37th Cong., 1st sess., *Senate Miscellaneous Document No. 2* (July 12, 1861).

"Mechanical and Other Employments for Patients in the British Lunatic Asylums." *American Journal of Insanity*, XIX (October 1862), 129–46.

"Sanitary Condition of the Army." *Atlantic Monthly*, X (October 1862), 463–97.

"Annual Report of the Trustees." In Worcester State Lunatic Hospital, *Annual Report*, XXX (1862), 5–47.

Letters to the Surgeon-General. In *Boston Medical and Surgical Journal*, LXVII (December 4, 1862), 363–67; (December 11, 1862), 381–84; LXVIII (April 9, 1863), 206.

"Annual Report of the Trustees." In Worcester State Lunatic Hospital, *Annual Report*, XXXI (1863), 3–36.

[Edward Jarvis et al.]. "Memorial [of the Trustees of the Worcester Lunatic Hospital]." Mass. *House Document No. 1* (January 1865).

"Influence of Distance From and Nearness to an Insane Hospital on its Use by the People." *American Journal of Insanity*, XXII (January 1866), 361–406.

"Connection of Intemperance with Disease and Mortality." *Boston Medical and Surgical Journal*, LXXIV (March 22, 1866), 149–54.

"Mortality Statistics . . . Eighth Census." In *Statistics of the United States, (Including Mortality, Property, &c.,) in 1860; Compiled from the Original Returns and Being the Final Exhibit of the Eighth Census.* Washington, D.C.: Government Printing Office, 1866. Pp. xxiii–lxvii, 1–287.

Testimony of Edward Jarvis. In *Reports on the Subject of a License Law, by a Joint Special Committee of the Legislature of Massachusetts; Together with a Stenographic Report of the Testimony Taken*

Before Said Committee. Boston: Wright & Potter, 1867. Also in
Mass. *House Document No. 415* (May 14, 1867).

"Director's Report." In Perkins Institution and Massachusetts Asylum
for the Blind, *Annual Report,* XXXVI (1867), 6–21.

[D. Humphreys Storer, Edward Jarvis, and Asa Millet]. "Memorial of
the Counsellors of the Massachusetts Medical Society." Mass. *House
Document No. 44* (1868).

Testimony of Edward Jarvis. In *Report of the Trial of Samuel M.
Andrews, Indicted for the Murder of Cornelius Holmes, before
the Supreme Judicial Court of Massachusetts, December 11, 1868*
(by Charles G. Davis). New York: Hurd and Houghton, 1869.

Letters to Congressman James A. Garfield. In *Communications from
Dr. Franklin B. Hough and Others, Relative to the Ninth Census of
the United States.* 41st Cong., 1st sess. *House Miscellaneous Document No. 33* (April 1, 1869), 27–42.

"Mania Transitoria." *Boston Medical and Surgical Journal,* n.s. III
(June 10, 1869), 329–37; (June 17, 1869), 353–57; also in
American Journal of Insanity, XXVI (July 1869), 1–32.

"Trial of Samuel M. Andrews for Murder." *Boston Medical and Sur-
gical Journal,* n.s. IV (November 4, 1869), 237–45; also appeared as
"Trial of Samuel M. Andrews for the Murder of Cornelius Holmes,"
American Journal of Insanity, XXVI (April 1870), 385–407.

"The Increase of Human Life." *Atlantic Monthly,* XXIV (October
1869), 495–506; (November 1869), 581–91; (December 1869),
711–18.

"A Memoir of John Conolly, M.D., D.C.L." *American Journal of
Insanity,* XXVI (April 1870), 470–85.

"Report of the Committee on Statistical Tables." *American Journal of
Insanity,* XXVIII (October 1871), 280–319.

"Proper Provision for the Insane." Mass. State Board of Health, *Annual Report,* III (1871), 139–59.

"Relation of Education and Insanity." In *Report of the Commissioner
of Education for the Year 1871.* Washington, D.C.: Government
Printing Office, 1872. Pp. 538–46.

"Ventilation of Dwellings and Sick Rooms." *Boston Medical and Surgical Journal,* n.s. IX (March 7, 1872), 149–51.

"Immigration." *Atlantic Monthly,* XXIX (April 1872), 454–68.

"Infant Mortality." Mass. State Board of Health, *Annual Report,* IV
(1872), 193–233.

"The Value of Common-School Education to Common Labor." In
Report of the Commissioner of Education for the Year 1872. Washington, D.C.: Government Printing Office, 1873. Pp. 572–85. Also

reprinted in U.S. Bureau of Education, *Circulars of Information,* no. 3 (1879). Washington, D.C.: Government Printing Office, 1879. Pp. 215–51.

"Political Economy of Health." Mass. State Board of Health, *Annual Report,* V (1873), 333–90.

"History of the Progress of Population of the United States of North America." In *Congrès International de Statistique, Compte-Rendu de la Huitième Session a St-Pétersbourg.* 3 vols. St-Pétersbourg: Imprimerie Trenke & Fusnot, 1874. Vol. III, 1–9. Also printed as pamphlet entitled *History of the Progress of Population of the United States. From 1790 to 1870.* Boston: David Clapp & Son, 1877.

"Vital Statistics of Different Races." *Journal of Social Science,* VII (September 1874), 229–34.

Letters to Dr. Henry I. Bowditch, March 6, November 20, 1876. In Henry I. Bowditch, *Public Hygiene in America.* Boston: Little, Brown, and Company, 1877. Pp. 172–74.

Letter to Henry J. Hosmer, March 16, 1882. In *The Centennial of the Social Circle in Concord March 21, 1882.* Cambridge: The Riverside Press, 1882.

Financial Connection of the Use of Spirits and Wine with the People of Concord, Massachusetts. Boston: T. Todd, 1883.

"The Supposed Decay of Families." *New England Historical and Genealogical Register,* XXXVIII (October 1884), 385–95. Also reprinted as *Supposed Decay of Families in New England: Disproved by the Experience of the People of Concord, Mass.* Boston: David Clapp & Son, 1884.

"Cookery and Health." *Unitarian Review and Religious Magazine,* XXII (November 1884), 401–16.

Index